ADVANCE I

"As the authors so beautifully illustrate in this book, looking good and feeling good are intricately connected. From the inside out, the health of our bodies are reflected in the appearance of our skin, among other things. It also works from the outside in. I've seen this over and over in my own life and with my own clients. When we like how we look, we feel better and take better care of ourselves. The program outlined in *Secret to a Younger You* will help you tap into the power of feeling good in your own skin!"

TAMI STACKELHOUSE, *Founder International Fibromyalgia Coaching Institute IFCInstitute.com*

"This book is written by two brilliant ND's who I have worked closely with over the past 10 years. I have experienced both personal treatments from them and have sent patients to them as well, all with great results (I am a practicing Chiropractor in Portland, Oregon). There are a myriad of conditions you can use their injections therapies for, including skin restoration as described in this book. I am passionate about alternative treatments that don't involve pharmaceuticals and surgery (two things this country does way too much of) and am happy this book is now available so that I can share it with my patients who may be interested in boosting their confidence in a healthy, self-preserving way. This book is a smooth read, easy to understand,

and written from the heart by two women who truly care about the overall health of their patients. It is refreshing to know there are non-synthetic alternatives out there with little to no side effects, that does not support big pharma, and that paves the way to a healthier you, naturally!"

DR. GRETCHEN BLYSS, *Owner of Blyss Chiropractic*

"This enlightening book walks you through the steps to revitalize your aging skin (and body) in a natural way avoiding harmful side effects and it provides its readers with a number of examples of how these options have helped others. I've done some of the treatments and have seen significant results. The PRP treatment made my neck firmer and more youthful looking, ozone therapy greatly reduced the coloration of a dark scar I have on my face (you can hardly see it now), and Phosphatidylcholine (PC) therapy has reduced Shingles breakouts from once a month to once every couple of years. Amazing results!"

THERESA BRAKEBUSH, *Principal*
Consultant of Ravensview Financial Services

"So excited about this book! As someone who works in the world of image as a stylist looking younger is something all of my clients want. And without chemicals or Botox is a dream. I eat organic and am super careful about what I put on my skin, but life happens. They offer a wonderful solution to looking younger without the nasties!!! A must read!"

ALEXANDRA GREENWALT,
Author of Love What You Wear

"*Secret To A Younger You* gives you an excellent understanding in the latest science based treatments for healthy skin. This advanced approach to reversing the affects of aging and toxicity go far beyond facelifts, botox and expensive chemical creams – naturally, quickly and without harmful side effects. I especially enjoyed chapter 5 which included detailed information about ozone injections and how beneficial it is for your skin and overall health. As an ozone practitioner for 14 years in giving ozonated colonics, and having given over 20,000 sessions, I have seen the amazing results of ozone in people's lives, especially the effect for skin conditions. I am so thankful for the work of Dr. McMonagle and Dr. Bourgeois to write such an easy to understand and informative book. I have also seen the results of this incredible technique by Dr. McMonagle and can't wait to try it myself. I turn 50 this year, and it will be my birthday present to me. You will not hear about this technique and approach from your medspa, average naturopath or aesthetician. Dr. Shallenberger's forward is also an excellent testimony to the credibility and effectiveness of their clinical work and this remarkable book."

REBECCA HARDER, *Owner of Colon Care, LLC*

"What an amazing read—both simple to understand and extremely relevant in today's fast paced society! Consistent daily grinds and the pursuit of "climbing" the ladders of success often distract so many from truly taking care of themselves through intentional, healthy life choices. Instead, we grab what's available on the go, we follow old paths of quick fixes, and we expose ourselves to unnecessary risks—often paying the price later in our journey. These clear explanations of safe, natural and effective ways to improve one's health, look younger and feel rejuvenated are impactful and inviting! Evidenced in many patient stories, simply making a few small changes lays the path for more significant efforts motivated by our own witnessing of powerful results. Thank you for bringing these options to light for a society which desperately needs more healthy options."

BRAD WULF, *Realtor at Keller Williams*

Secret to a Younger YOU

SECRET
TO A
YOUNGER
YOU

The 3 Month Program:

A Natural Facelift Without Botox

Dr. Bridghid McMonagle &
Dr. Kaley Bourgeois

NEW YORK

LONDON • NASHVILLE • MELBOURNE • VANCOUVER

Secret to a Younger YOU

The 3 Month Program: A Natural Facelift Without Botox

Published in New York, New York, by Morgan James Publishing in partnership with Difference Press. Morgan James is a trademark of Morgan James, LLC. www.MorganJamesPublishing.com

The Morgan James Speakers Group can bring authors to your live event. For more information or to book an event visit The Morgan James Speakers Group at www.TheMorganJamesSpeakersGroup.com.

ISBN 9781683506799 paperback
ISBN 9781683506805 eBook
Library of Congress Control Number: 2017911521

Cover and Interior Design by:
Chris Treccani
www.3dogcreative.net

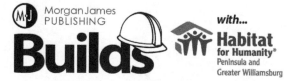

In an effort to support local communities, raise awareness and funds, Morgan James Publishing donates a percentage of all book sales for the life of each book to Habitat for Humanity Peninsula and Greater Williamsburg.

Get involved today! Visit
www.MorganJamesBuilds.com

Dedication

To all of our patients who allow us to be part of their ongoing journeys toward optimal health. We feel honored to be part of your process.

To those we meet during our own journey who inspire us to ask questions, challenge ourselves, and support safer medicine.

Primum Non Nocere

TABLE OF CONTENTS

FOREWORD

Everybody wants to look good. Well, on second thought let me correct that. Everybody wants to look like what they think looks good. But one thing I am pretty sure of is that nobody wants the wrinkles, saggy skin, pigmentations, and dull, lifeless skin that happens with aging. No one. So as these charming little evidences of our mortality show up, we try to do everything we can that is reasonable to get them to disappear. And the statistics bear this out.

Just in the United States alone we spend eight billion dollars every year on cosmetics (www.worldwatch.org/node/764). It's not just women spending this money. The guys are also in on the action. And that's not even counting any of the money spent on plastic surgery. So, here's the big question:

What if you could look better without simply covering things up with cosmetics? Young people don't need cosmetics. So, what if you could regain the glow and luster of the healthy skin you had in your youth? And here's an even better question.

What if by doing what you needed to do to look better, you actually were better? I mean better all over. What if your overall health inside improved just as much as your appearance outside? And that's what I like so much about this book. It tells you how to do just that.

Your skin is important. Leaving aside the issue of appearance, the skin is an organ just like any other organ. It performs many significant functions for your general health. The skin helps to regulate your temperature and your hydration status. Vitamin D is made in your skin. Your skin has special immune cells called dendritic cells that interact with your environment to protect you from toxins and infections. And so, anything you can do to improve your skin also improves your overall health and vitality. The same things that improve your skin, from hormones to vital nutrients to detoxification are also going to improve your liver, your heart, your brain, and everything else in between.

I like to look good. I'm definitely not against plastic surgery if that's what you need. But let's face it (pun intended), why would I want to spend all that money and risk the potential complications that can occur with any surgery if it only improves my appearance and doesn't do anything else for the rest of my body?

So, enjoy *Secret To A Younger You*. Follow the advice in this book and you will not only look better and younger, you will also feel and function better and younger. And from my perspective, that's what being healthy is all about.

FRANK SHALLENBERGER, *MD, HMD, FAAO,*
President, American Academy of Ozonotherapy,
Author of Bursting With Energy, The Principles and
Applications of Ozone Therapy, The Ozone Miracle,
and The Type 2 Diabetes Breakthrough

INTRODUCTION

Deciding whether to schedule cosmetic procedures is not always simple or easy. Surgeries, Botox and synthetic fillers can come with a large price tag, painful recovery time, and often dramatic outcomes that may be good or bad. If you found our book, none of this is news to you. You know the struggle well. *I don't like these lines, but can I afford a facelift?* You probably can, but there may be other reasons you hesitate. *I always look like I'm frowning, but do I want to look frozen from Botox?* Looking different can be just as unsettling as looking older. Finding a balance between erasing years and creating a new look may seem daunting.

The social stigma around cosmetic procedures is just as conflicting. After all, friends, family and even strangers often share opinions about the "right" way to take care of yourself and how to build your self-esteem. Even if you feel secure in your values, the judgments of others can take a toll. The possibility of looking different, rather than younger and healthier, adds to this concern. As doctors, we know there is no shame in taking care of your skin, and even if you feel the same, you still face social pressures.

Maybe you are concerned about the risks of allergic reaction and want to avoid injecting toxins and preservatives. If so, Botox and synthetic fillers are not for you. That doesn't mean you can't reduce wrinkles and improve the quality of your skin without surgery. We wrote this book to tell you *there is a way to look and feel younger without scheduling Botox or surgery*.

Remember, the skin on your face matters. It works hard to share your expressions and communicate your emotions and thoughts. Your skin is also a sign of your health seen by everyone you meet. You deserve to feel proud of the face you present to the world, and we can help you nurture that pride without the fear of surgery or toxins.

The positive impact of minor cosmetic procedures on self-esteem is well documented in research. One such study tracked a group of adults for six months following minimally invasive procedures and found that the majority reported better self-esteem and better quality of life [1].

You instinctually know that improving your appearance will benefit your quality of life, otherwise you would not be considering cosmetic medicine. *How* it benefits you depends on your individual values, goals and feelings. Most often, it depends on what you *aren't* doing because of your insecurities. Cosmetic medicine, or aesthetic medicine, is a rapidly growing field in the United States. These terms encompass a variety of techniques used to improve your appearance. In our book, we are focusing on improving fine lines and wrinkles as well as your hair. We also include a method used to improve cellulite and scars. This is done via injections, intravenous treatments, nutritional changes, and more.

As you read this book you will become acquainted with many of our patients who faced the same conflicts you may be experiencing. Though we changed their names, their health struggles and decision to try cosmetic medicine are as real as yours. We want to introduce you to Debbie first, because her health story is very similar to so many of our other patients' experiences. When Debbie first came to our clinic, she scheduled for our natural cosmetic facial injections. She was 51 years old with a few general health complaints that were bothering her, but overall healthy and excited to look younger. Like so many of our patients, Debbie came in for one specific concern (wrinkles), but ended up inspired to make bigger health changes. We focused on the "stupid lines" as she called them, starting with injections. While decreasing her fine lines and wrinkles didn't directly improve her other health complaints, such as hot flashes and joint pain, Debbie told us she felt more motivated to try additional things which might. Sometimes improving quality of life through enhancing appearance has a positive effect on self-esteem and overall motivation to work on other health concerns.

Debbie became a realtor in her early 40s and noticed that first impressions count. When she saw more opportunities going to younger women in her real estate group, she became concerned that her age might be a factor. Did improving her appearance boost Debbie's self-confidence? Of course it did. Did fewer lines attract more clients? Probably not, but the new way she carried herself and her visible self-confidence likely did.

Whether you want to boost general self-confidence or you have a specific goal such as improving your work performance or dating again, you *deserve* to enhance your quality of life. We will help you do that without surgery, toxins or synthetic fillers.

"Your body is a temple, but only if you treat it as one."

~Astrid Alauda

CHAPTER 1

Age Gracefully

At this point, you may be wondering who we are and what motivates us to offer an alternative to standard cosmetic medicine procedures. How did we become inspired to learn a more natural injection technique, and what led us to prioritize a whole-body approach?

We are both licensed Naturopathic Physicians in Oregon, where we've built a thriving practice. Each of us enjoys focusing on functional and regenerative medicine in addition to cosmetic procedures. We dedicated ourselves to the service of treating the whole person when we chose this career. This includes anything that contributes to physical and emotional health. Most certainly, this includes any concerns that impact self-esteem.

Many Naturopathic Physicians offer Botox, Juvederm, Restyline and other "standard" cosmetic procedures. It's a lucrative business, as these products offer immediate results. We decided early on that we would rather offer a non-toxic cosmetic procedure that can reduce fine lines and wrinkles without adding to an individual's toxic burden. Toxic burden refers to the bioaccumulation of synthetic and natural compounds that weigh heavily on a body's ability to detoxify. Impacts of such accumulation vary with each individual. There can be negative changes seen in every system of the body, including immune system and reproductive function [2].

Although preservatives and additives found in the products mentioned above contribute only a small amount to one's toxic burden, our goal is to reduce those exposures wherever possible. The environment is laden with chemical preservatives, pesticides, heavy metals and other toxins. Many of these are man-made, others are naturally occurring. How much we are each exposed to matters, and we strive to serve our patients by offering therapies that don't add to the burden.

Sometimes chemical exposures are necessary when the benefits are greater than the risks. This is the decision we make each time we take an antibiotic or a blood pressure medication. The liver must work harder to process these chemicals, and there may be other consequences such as changes in the microflora of the gut. We should evaluate risks when we consider cosmetic procedures as well. Since we offer an effective alternative for our patients, they can choose an option with fewer risks and still see wonderful outcomes.

As doctors, we don't just want your skin to look healthier, we want it to *be* healthier. Now that we've explained why we offer something different, we want to individually share with you why we are passionate about cosmetic medicine.

A Note from Dr. Bridghid McMonagle

When I first began working in medicine, I admit that I had a negative perspective of cosmetic procedures. I was attached to the idea that they represented vanity, which was not a value I wanted to emphasize in my patients or myself. Often I saw a lack of expression in my patients after multiple injections or surgeries and I was concerned they would take it too far. I did not want to contribute to that, especially in my patients who seemed unhappy with how they looked no matter what they changed.

I recall the exact patient who showed me that my initial aversion to cosmetic medicine was not needed. A few years into practice, a female patient of mine showed a dramatic turn around in her self-confidence and her daily health choices. For her, that shift didn't happen easily, and it didn't happen until she began feeling more attractive. We worked for months on nutrition, diet recommendations and other basic health support. She made some changes, but wasn't motivated to maintain any of them.

It was after we completed an intense, 4-week weight loss program which provided quick results that things began to change. After losing 28 pounds, even though the diet program was over and everything went back to "normal," her motivation changed. My bias toward cosmetic medicine changed as well. As a result of the weight loss, she felt more attractive, and as it turns out, more motivated to create further changes. She was less shy about going to the gym, which helped with further weight loss and fitness gains. Her excitement led to her feeling ready for long-term diet changes, and I also noticed her making more eye contact than before. Now she wanted to work on the appearance of her face. She didn't like that her lines were more visible since her weight loss. I had no problem supporting this. I knew she was on a great path now. This is when I realized that cosmetic procedures weren't really about vanity. For many people, looking better can create the motivation to do things that make them feel better. An external change can be the motivation for an internal change. For this patient, it started with weight loss but for many, it starts with presenting a more youthful look to others. Whatever it is, as long as it is safe, I like to support that journey. It brings me a lot of joy to see patients come in for cosmetic reasons and leave with the knowledge it takes to continue improvements in their skin and overall health.

A Note from Dr. Kaley Bourgeois

My passion for cosmetic medicine, and specifically natural cosmetic medicine, came about through experiences I had with loved ones. When I first opened my practice, I did not foresee focusing on aesthetic procedures. It was not that I had an aversion to this corner of the health industry. In fact, I always saw myself as someone with a general appreciation of medical aesthetics.

Like many Americans, I have more than one family member who uses cosmetic procedures in an effort to restore or improve their appearance. I value the insight this provides me, both into their process for deciding what to do, and more importantly, the emotional and social concerns they experience. Self-esteem and confidence are always the first thing mentioned when we discuss their cosmetic treatments. Fear of social scrutiny also comes up. What I've learned through family members reveals a clear pattern: They are mostly worried about upsetting the ideals and expectations of their loved ones, and less conflicted over their own feelings about cosmetic procedures.

One notable experience was a minor surgical complication experienced by a family member that eventually inspired me to invest myself in natural procedures. The procedure, a brow lift, resulted in nerve damage and daily shooting pains that did not fade as hoped. Is it tolerable? Yes. Is it minor as surgical complications go? Absolutely. But maybe it wasn't necessary. They felt limited in their options, and didn't see an alternative to Botox or surgery. Being able to offer such an alternative gave rise to my passion for cosmetic medicine.

CHAPTER 2

The 3 Month Program Made For You

You probably have concerns and questions about cosmetic procedures. Maybe you've even had Botox or surgery in the past and you realized you want something different this time. Making the decision to try something new can be both exciting and a bit frightening. Understanding your options will help you decide the right route for your cosmetic support. Which procedure will look most natural? Are you worried about embarrassment if people can see you've had work done? Questions about the safety of cosmetic procedures are equally important, including allergic reactions and other complications.

Cosmetic surgery can go wrong. It may result in large, visible scars or an uneven appearance. Botox may leave you with a headache, flu-like symptoms or asymmetrical features like a droopy eyelid. These side effects may resolve, but is it worth the risk if there is a safer alternative? It is possible to experience botulism effects systemically, as well. This can present as muscle weakness, trouble swallowing and even difficulty breathing. These are not benign problems to face.

The product insert for Botox includes:

"WARNING: DISTANT SPREAD OF TOXIN EFFECT Post marketing reports indicate that the effects of BOTOX Cosmetic and all botulinum toxin products may spread from the area of injection to produce symptoms consistent with botulinum toxin effects. These may include asthenia, generalized muscle weakness, diplopia, ptosis, dysphagia, dysphonia, dysarthria, urinary incontinence and breathing difficulties. These symptoms have been reported hours to weeks after injection. Swallowing and breathing difficulties can be life threatening and there have been reports of death. The risk of symptoms is probably greatest in children treated for spasticity but symptoms can also occur in adults treated for spasticity and other conditions, particularly in those patients who have an underlying condition that would predispose them to these symptoms. In unapproved uses, including spasticity in children, and in approved indications, cases of spread of effect have been

reported at doses comparable to those used to treat cervical dystonia and upper limb spasticity and at lower doses."

*"**Cardiovascular System** There have been reports following administration of BOTOX of adverse events involving the cardiovascular system, including arrhythmia and myocardial infarction, some with fatal outcomes. Some of these patients had risk factors including pre-existing cardiovascular disease. Use caution when administering to patients with pre-existing cardiovascular disease."*

You want to feel better about how you look without feeling guilty for that desire. You are not alone, as statistics demonstrate. According to the American Society of Plastic Surgeons, in 2015 there were 6.7 million Botox procedures, 2.4 million fillers and 1.3 million chemical peels. In the US, 49% of the cosmetic procedures performed were for women between 40-54 years old. A staggering $13.3 billion was spent and an increasing amount of procedures are being offered in office-based settings. Cosmetic procedures for men are also on the rise.

We know that when you look and feel better, your confidence and self-esteem will improve. Providing that change with fewer concerns about toxicity or unsightly scars was part of the motivation for creating our program. This book will outline how we combine natural cosmetic injections with nutritional, diet and lifestyle changes to enhance the anti-aging effects.

Through this program, you will learn how to take better care of your skin and see lasting improvement. You will learn how to protect your skin from damage by changing daily routines and switching to superior topical treatments that are affordable, researched and actually work. We will discuss how food can affect your skin, and how to make diet changes. Do you think eating gluten-free is too trendy? Maybe it is just another fad? We will dive into the role this might play in your skin's appearance, as well as discussing other effective diet changes for skin health. If you suffer from adult acne or other inflammatory skin disorders, you will learn solutions to your problems. We also utilize systemic therapies, such as intravenous treatments, that have research demonstrating anti-aging effects and other skin benefits. The program includes options for hormone testing and support to further enhance your results.

You will want to read this book before you call the office to schedule your new patient visit so that you know what to expect. We also offer two webinars to help you get started. The webinars will give you guidance to start implementing change now so you don't have to wait for your initial appointment.

There are a few things our clinic staff will discuss with you over the phone to make sure you have everything you need to get started before your first visit. Basic screening labs are needed before procedures can be initiated, whether ordered through your current primary care physician (PCP) or with us. We require basic screening labs not older than three months.

If this is not possible, we can arrange them during your first appointment. When you become a member of this program, we do not take the place of your PCP. We recommend all our cosmetic medicine patients maintain regular care with labs and physical exam through a general practitioner. During your hour-long new patient visit, we will assess your individual skin needs, recommend specific labs if any are indicated, confirm your schedule for treatments and get you started on your path to minimizing lines!

The facial injections are scheduled four weeks apart, one session per month. Intravenous therapies can be scheduled for the day preceding or following injections, and you will receive a daily oral and topical skin support regimen for home use. At the end of the 3-month program, we include a follow-up visit to discuss long-term goals and develop your maintenance protocol. This includes a custom prescription facial cream, personalized CD34/PRP facial serum (discussed more in Chapter 7), and options for additional lab screenings and support. For lasting results, our patients follow up once a year for maintenance injections. As needed, we do modify the maintenance program. When you schedule your new patient appointment, we will provide you with a list of places you can stay if traveling, and we will schedule you for each of your treatments.

As with any procedure, there are risks. Our new patient paperwork includes a list of contraindications and addresses safety concerns. These documents are provided electronically along with a copy of your scheduled appointments and an additional form where you can highlight those areas of your skin that are your highest priority. We will need to be alerted of any drug allergies prior to your appointment.

After the first procedure is completed, which takes approximately 1 hour, you will notice that the areas where we used a natural filler are not as pronounced. Redness generally resolves within 24-48 hours, and there may be some mild bruising that warrants foundation or concealer for one to two weeks. Over the next few months of treatment, you will notice your skin appears brighter and fuller, depth of wrinkles lessen, and treated areas of discoloration may fade. Patients report the pain as mild and easy to tolerate. We use a prescription numbing cream to minimize discomfort from the needles. Rather than introduce synthetic chemicals and toxins to temporarily restore the appearance of youthful skin, our approach stimulates your skin's production of collagen. This results in skin that is acutally healthier. If you want a safer, effective way to enhance your beauty and confidence, this is the program for you.

CHAPTER 3

Your Lines Are Unique & So Are Your Needs

When Becky first showed up in our clinic, she was only 38 and already had an impressive collection of creams. Although she scheduled her visit to discuss years of eczema, she mentioned also struggling with rosacea and ingrown hairs. During her first physical, we discovered those ingrown hairs were actually an inflammatory rash called hidradenitis suppurativa. She also told us she thought her rosacea was acne at first. Why did it matter if Becky had acne or rosacea? Ingrown hairs or hidradenitis suppurativa? It mattered because skin is not simple. A rash on two different people may look the same, but have different diagnoses. Likewise, wrinkles appear similar on all of us, but we don't all respond to the same creams. For Becky, mistaking her rosacea for acne led to several years of irritating acne creams and sadly, tanning. The "acne" didn't go away, and she developed new fine lines around her eyes. As for the painful bumps under her arms, no amount of scrubbing, waxing or "au natural" helped because she was treating the wrong condition.

Like Becky, you want to understand your skin and you want to see it improve. The good news is it's not too late to start. After all, your skin is always renewing. Stem cells continuously give rise to a new epidermis, the outer layer that you see and feel. Even though this process slows in middle age, it's as if you have a new face every month [3]. Deeper lines and rashes may take more time to respond to treatments, but they do respond.

Remember Debbie? Her skin wasn't renewing as fast at 51 years old as it did when she was 20. She noticed small cuts and bruises took a bit longer to heal and wondered if she needed a multivitamin. This is one of the first things she mentioned at her new patient visit. We included nutritional support in Debbie's treatment, and we also discussed aging and skin turnover. Natural, lasting improvements like we see with our cosmetic injections take time since we are creating change in the health and integrity of the skin itself. A quick fix like Botox is satisfying at first, but the benefits are short-lived. This was part of why Debbie came for something different, and she later told us she felt better about that decision after she began learning about her skin.

Slower skin regeneration isn't the only thing that gradually decreases the youthfulness of your face. The repetitive expressions you make every day contribute, too. If you smile often, you'll have more prominent smile lines. Likewise, if you frown for hours on end, those frown lines will eventually stick. The emotions you wear are not the only cause of your wrinkles, but over time, they will determine which stand out most prominently [4] Are you squinting constantly at a computer screen, deepening an already furrowed brow? Are you wearing work frustrations on your face? Muscle retraining techniques to even out lines are popular because expressions play a role [5].

The basic anatomy of your skin is never more than a few clicks away with today's internet. The biological workings of this extensive organ are impressive, from the outermost epidermis, to the collagen-filled middle layer named the dermis, and finally the deeper hypodermis that is rich in fat. All of your skin layers play a role in the development of lines. What interests us, and hopefully you as well, are specific details about what keeps these layers firm, including which nutrients the cells need most.

In this chapter, we will focus specifically on fibroblasts, collagen, elastin, moisture and vital nutrients. Fibroblasts are a type of connective tissue cell that lives in your dermis, the middle layer we mentioned above. These busy cells are responsible for producing collagen. The health and density of your collagen, types I and III to be exact, determines how firm your skin looks and feels. Elastin is an equally important connective tissue protein, also made by fibroblasts. Elastin helps your skin hold its shape. Think of it as the rubber band in your skin. When it stretches, elastin pulls it back into place [6].

As skin ages, production of both collagen and elastin decreases. This means your body is slower to replace old connective tissue with new connective tissue, even though the rate of breakdown isn't slowing. In fact, cumulative years of sun damage and other environmental factors may result in a faster rate of breakdown. As a result, the skin is less firm, less elastic, and less youthful.

Moisture in the upper layer, the epidermis, also decreases with age. This results from a variety of factors, including decreased production of moisturizing substances from the keratinocytes (cells) in the upper layer as well as decreased hormones. As estrogen and testosterone decrease in both men and women, skin produces less oil and struggles to hold moisture. Dry skin appears less full and accentuates lines. It is helpful to understand this general decline in hormones that comes with aging, but hormone changes will vary from person to person. For this reason, the hormonal changes you see in your skin will come at different ages for everyone. Some men and women may even experience acne and oily skin later in life. These differences are why it is so important to understand your skin and look at what underlies it.

Supporting the health and growth of your connective tissue relies on key nutrients. Most of these nutrients are obtained through a healthy diet, but increasing specific food groups and supplementing is important when trying to optimize tissue regeneration. Also, digestion and absorption can slow as we age, making supplementation even more important. One example is amino acids, the tiny building blocks of proteins. These are essential for production of collagen and elastin, as well as the moisturizing substances in the epidermis. Often we supplement these building blocks while working on digestive health so that you are better able to derive them from food in coming years. Vitamin C is also essential for a healthy epidermis. It protects skin by serving as an antioxidant, and it directly stimulates increased collagen production [7]. We will discuss diet and supplementation in depth during a later chapter.

We've established your skin's innate ability to regenerate, but what about the impact of external factors and everyday stressors on that process? Certain internal factors, like genetics, are beyond our control. We prefer to focus on what we can change. This includes sun exposure, repetitive expressions, stress, poor sleep, bad digestion, poor nutrition, hormone imbalances and inflammatory conditions.

It is well established that UV radiation via sun exposure speeds up aging through the breakdown of collagen [8]. Tanning beds have the same effect, which Becky experienced while trying to treat what she thought was acne. Your body's reliance upon

UV to produce vitamin D is just one of many reasons time in direct sunshine is beneficial, so we do not recommend strict UV avoidance. However, protecting sensitive areas such as your face is appropriate, especially if you live in areas of increased UV exposure. By the time Becky came to us, she was no longer tanning, but the wrinkles were getting deeper. At 43, her lines were fine and easy to treat. We were able to reduce their depth and give her skin a firmer appearance with three sessions of platelet rich plasma injections.

Stress and poor sleep both contribute to the aging process, and it can show on your face. Chronic stress results in hormone imbalances that elevate blood sugar and contribute to oxidative damage throughout the body. Our bodies perform a continual dance between oxidative and antioxidant processes. Both are necessary in our physiology, but too much unbalanced oxidation interrupts skin regeneration and health. Our gender hormones, including estrogen and testosterone, are also important for skin health and maintenance. Though these are not stress hormones, they are sensitive to our mental and emotional states. Sleep deprivation, natural aging processes, chronic infections, and environmental toxins all contribute to hormone imbalances that impact our skin. Sleep deprivation can elevate stress hormones, but there is the additional concern of mechanical compression leading to asymmetrical lines and wrinkles over time [9]. In other words, always sleeping on one side of your face can cause asymmetry.

Chronic stress can also disrupt digestion, leading to changes in the delicate ecosystem contained within your gut. It may seem as though skin and digestion are separate, and perhaps a prior physician told you as much. Clinically, we see that there is a clear connection. Skin and digestive health cannot be separated. Irritation in the gut, whether from dysbiosis (an imbalance between good and bad bacteria), food intolerances or an Inflammatory Bowel Disease, leads to signs of inflammation in the skin.

When we treat the gut in our patients, their skin shows positive changes. These changes include better moisture, fewer inflammatory rashes such as eczema, psoriasis or acne, and less unsightly swelling around the eyes. Modern science has shown us how much impact your microbiome (your gut's own individualized ecosystem) has on immune function and health so it should not be surprising that changes to digestion equate to changes in skin health. This is another reason why nutrients, and especially diet, cannot be overlooked in anti-aging medicine. Certain foods may irritate the gut and increase your risk for digestive disorders. Likewise, certain digestive disorders will interrupt your ability to properly break down meals and absorb nutrients needed by your skin.

What is the significance of inflammatory conditions like Becky's? These include rosacea, eczema, hidradenitis suppurativa and numerous others. A patch of eczema does not directly age skin in the same way as UV exposure or hormone deficiencies, but it does indicate a pattern of generalized inflammation. Chronic inflammation interrupts your ability to heal and regenerate. This affects every tissue in your body, skin included.

In Becky's case, her rashes responded well to anti-inflammatory therapies. It was not enough to simply prescribe a steroid or antibiotic cream. She had those in the past for her eczema, and the results were never lasting. We worked together to develop targeted dietary changes, introduce an individualized regimen of nutrients, and choose non-toxic topical ointments. With the right diet and anti-inflammatory support, Becky saw lasting improvement.

Like Becky, your skin and overall health are unique to you. You see these individual traits every day in the form of a specific smile line, sometimes a new rash or hair loss when you are stressed. You and your skin have a close relationship, so you've probably picked up on a few of the foods or activities that impact it. Part of our approach to help you look and feel younger includes enhancing this relationship, by working with you to take a closer look at what impacts your skin every day.

CHAPTER 4

Loving My New Face!

Before Debbie scheduled with us, she heard about platelet rich plasma (PRP) cosmetic injections from a friend. It sounded too good to be true and she told us she felt skeptical at first. Debbie also hated needles, so anything that included injections scared her. Still feeling intrigued, she did some research online and on our website. Her friend told her it wasn't as painful as she might think. After only a week, Debbie called us, ready to schedule.

At her first visit, Debbie explained how she tried Botox once. As she was talking, we noticed she avoided eye contact. It seemed she was embarrassed about it, which she later confirmed. She didn't want to look like the expressionless people she sometimes noticed. Debbie wanted to feel good about her choice and feel

21

confident talking about her decisions with her friends. She was also very nervous about pain and recovery time. Debbie recounted how painful the Botox injections were. Her hands would sweat at the thought of them. We took time to discuss the procedure in detail with her. The needles are very small, the solution is prepared in a way that it is virtually pain free, and the injections are not deep. At the end of the appointment, we had her watch a video of the procedure. This calmed her immediately. On the video, the client was not flinching with any of the needle sticks. She was excited to get started.

During the next few months, Debbie opened up more about her physical and emotional health concerns. We often see this happening. We have patients who don't want to go to the gym until they lose weight, or those who are recently divorced and don't feel confident enough to date. As they work on their roadblocks to health, their whole life changes. Sometimes, it can be as simple as starting with reducing fine lines. Debbie mentioned that her eczema, even though virtually gone after working with us, left discoloration on her forearms and her neck. She inquired if the cosmetic PRP could work on this too. After a few sessions of local injections, discoloration faded and the skin started to appear normal again. Her skin wasn't bad after the diet changes and treatments, but it was another piece of the puzzle that was limiting her self-confidence.

Another patient, Jenny, scheduled after seeing before and after pictures on our website. Initially, she felt frustrated. Why didn't she know there was a natural option for wrinkles that worked? The Botox she got 6 months ago got rid of her lines, but it also changed her expressions. Now those results were gone. It seemed like a waste of money. Frustration turned to curiosity and eventually excitement. She called and had her first set of injections performed a month later at our clinic. She felt better about telling her friends that her fuller skin was treated with her own platelets rather than Botox. She also liked that no one asked her if she got Botox, like they did before.

Why don't more Americans know about these natural alternatives to Botox and fillers, known as platelet rich plasma injections (PRP)? PRP injections use your own platelets from your blood to safely stimulate new collagen growth. These can be used in areas of wrinkles, sagging skin, and thinning hair. We met a boutique owner from Peru who knew all about this therapy. Her mom used it for decades. We've met more individuals like this, living outside of the USA, that are better versed in effective alternative cosmetic medicine than many of our local patients, friends and family. If your prior physicians and estheticians didn't tell you about it, it's likely because they've never heard of PRP therapy.

PRP therapy was first used medically in the USA during the 1970s. After a blood draw in our office, we use a centrifuge to separate out part of your blood, add a few nutrients, and prepare your cosmetic injectable. Your platelets start releasing growth factors within 10 minutes of their preparation. They can help to even skin tone, minimize scars, clear up acne, improve loose skin, and diminish fine lines. We continually update our procedures and instruments to ensure optimal results. One of the methods we utilize at our clinic is prepping part of your platelets with a specialized heater that makes a natural filler. The natural filler can give immediate results, while the PRP takes a bit longer. We have added a list of resources at the end of the book which you can visit for additional information and research.

Fine lines disappear over time following the procedure, and the needling itself helps to stimulate stem cells and healing aspects just under your skin. Depending on your skin, we may recommend additional nutrients added to this combination. We provide a thorough evaluation at your first visit to ensure your needs are met. In addition to providing our perspective on areas that may benefit from injections, we take time to listen to what really bothers you. For some people it is the crease between their eyebrows that makes them feel like they look angry in photos. For others, it is the smile lines that don't go away. There may be some sagging to your skin along your jawline that you would like to work on or perhaps dark circles around your eyes. Your priority is our priority.

With a client around 25-35 years old who has finer lines, we can use PRP with no filler or additional nutrients. In clients with more advanced signs of aging, we add powerful tools to enhance the results. These may include vitamin C to aid in collagen production, and hyaluronic acid which is a natural substance in your extracellular matrix that acts as a cushion. That cushion decreases with age. Hyaluronic acid can be added to the injections to help improve the volume in your skin and decrease thinning. This is also part of the cushion that shrinks in our joints and worsens with over-the-counter pain killers such as aspirin [10].

Missy was in her 60s when she came to us. Her husband recently left her for a younger woman. She was feeling insecure about the thought of dating for the first time in 30 years and wanted to lose about 15 pounds. Her joints ached and she didn't like what she saw in the mirror. Her friend told her about what we offer at the clinic and she was intrigued. The cosmetic procedures we performed over the next 3 months. She noticed healthier looking skin and felt her confidence returning. Soon after the treatments, she purchased a gym membership. In 4 months she lost 25 pounds. This process snowballed into a path of healing and happiness for Missy. This is what we love to witness.

As patients are reminded of who they were, and how they felt when they were younger, they are motivated to make healthy lifestyle changes. We often see men and women become more consistent with diet changes, more assertive at work, and overall more confident. Others are drawn to this newfound confidence.

Medical ozone gas is used along with PRP injections, both to enhance the platelets in the plasma itself, and as a stand-alone injectable medicine. Studies indicate that ozone therapy improves oxygen delivery to tissues, increases growth factors and stem cells, improves release of nitric oxide (NO), which increases circulation, and stimulates our natural antioxidant processes. Ozone therapy can also be used to reduce the appearance of cellulite, aid in fat breakdown, improve skin tone, minimize scarring, and enhance tissue healing. When we first learned about ozone therapy, it was rarely mentioned in medical school. Through continued medical training, we both became fascinated by the healing properties of ozone in combination with PRP.

Medical uses for ozone gas first arose in the 1800s. The majority of us think about ozone as a form of pollution, contributing to respiratory ailments. Some people are familiar with air purifiers that emit very small amounts of ozone to clean the air. The use of medical ozone is much different. Ozone is made from oxygen tanks attached to a medical grade ozone generator that delivers a clean combination of oxygen ($O2$) and ozone ($O3$), used for various medical conditions. It can be injected directly into joints, cellulite and other tissues. It can also be added to certain intravenous therapies for systemic benefits. Neither of us can imagine practicing without these powerful, natural therapies. Our patients travel from all over the states and internationally to take advantage of these treatments. We included several research article links at the back of this book if you would like to learn more.

Another patient, Sarah, was always told she looked young for her age and had perfect skin. She recently had a bout of acne during a stressful phase of her life that scarred in several places. She didn't like wearing foundation, but felt she had to cover up the scarring. Sarah felt silly at the gym and outdoor activities with makeup on. After a few injections of both platelets and medical ozone, her scars faded so much she didn't even notice them. Sarah was overjoyed to have her skin back.

PRP therapy and the cosmetic use of ozone are becoming highly sought after methods to achieve cosmetic improvements and avoid the surgical knife. How long do you have to wait to see results? When filler is used, only an hour. How long do they last? We see improvements even one year after the injections. With so much potential benefit and the significant reduction in risk for allergic reaction and unnecessary binders and preservatives, it's no surprise that this alternative is gaining popularity.

CHAPTER 5

How Can Intravenous Therapies Help My Skin?

Denise was in her 50s when she came to see us, not long after being diagnosed with Fibromyalgia. She worried about "letting herself go," but said it was hard to care when she had so much muscle and joint pain. She appeared much older than she was, and felt sad recalling how she was a professional ballet dancer in her prime. She found us while searching for ozone therapy after hearing it could help her body pain. Her muscle aches were gone after three intravenous (IV) treatments using ozone, and her joint pain was considerably better following two sessions of joint injections. When Denise started feeling better, she asked about treatments for her wrinkles. She had a new lease on life and was ready to see more positive change.

The IVs Denise had for pain can also help with skin health, which she noticed when her rosacea started to clear up. We routinely prescribe these IVs as part of the protocol for skin regeneration because the results are much more impressive. Usually the patients getting IVs with their facial injections notice more than just skin changes. This was the case with Debbie. She had an IV treatment with ozone after every session, and following her second IV, mentioned that her fatigue was gone. What fatigue? At her first visit, Debbie told us her energy was "normal." It turned out that Debbie's new normal was actually different from how she felt for years prior when we met her. Until she had better energy, she didn't even realize how tired she'd become.

At this point, you are probably wondering what we are talking about when we mention Ozone IVs. IV Medical Ozone therapy, better known as Major Autohemotherapy (MAH), has been used since the 1800s. There are many names that refer to this treatment depending on what country you are in, or where a particular research article was created. In addition to IV Medical Ozone therapy and MAH, you may also see it called Autohemotherapy (AHT), autologous therapy, immune modulation, and immunotherapy. We will refer to it in this book as MAH. MAH is a simple and effective therapy. A small volume of blood is withdrawn and safely mixed with a combination of ozone and oxygen. The medical grade ozone reacts with your red blood cells immediately, at which time your blood becomes bright red. This indicates that it is highly oxygenated. The gas is dissolved and your blood can then be safely returned to you.

This is a comfortable and relaxing treatment. Most patients describe a sense of general wellbeing during the treatment. Others describe their breathing as easier, and some of our patients comment that their vision seems sharper. The most common response to the IV is leaving the clinic feeling better than when you walked in. Minor illnesses typically resolve quickly, so this is a popular IV during cold and flu season.

Jenna came in for MAH treatments to address daily fatigue. She told us afterward that the results were amazing. She felt she had her full energy back after 6 treatments. Jenna never mentioned she also had daily abdominal pain. She was diagnosed with Irritable Bowel Syndrome and had given up on trying different medications and supplements to decrease the cramping and discomfort. After the first ozone treatment, her abdominal pain was gone. We don't know exactly why it resolved, but Jenna didn't care. She also noticed that her skin seemed clearer, less ruddy.

Medical ozone, when used via IV, causes many reactions in our bodies that are beneficial to our health. We have mentioned some before. Here is a more comprehensive list of benefits:

- Improved oxygenation of tissues
- Flexible red blood cells that can more easily travel through your smallest blood vessels
- Stimulation of growth factors
- Decreased inflammation
- Enhanced detoxification
- Faster wound healing
- Increased antioxidant enzyme activity
- General anti-aging benefits

There are other ways to take advantage of medical ozone therapy that do not require needles or good veins. We have several options if MAH is not for you or we are not able to perform that procedure due to very small veins. Don't worry, we will make sure you can receive the benefits of ozone therapy.

Another IV therapy that has several amazing healing properties is Glutathione. Glutathione is made up of three amino acids: cysteine, glycine and glutamate.

There are many benefits to these IVs, including:

- Powerful anti-oxidant action
- Major support for detoxification pathways
- Skin-lightening benefits
- Energy improvement

Brenda is one of our patients who swears by glutathione IV therapy. When she noticed mild tremors in her hands, she became concerned. Multiple sclerosis and other worrisome neurological conditions were ruled out by her neurologist, but she still felt unwell. Her walking seemed off, not as stable, and the tremors were daily. She stopped scheduling outings with friends, and after thinking about it, realized it was mostly due to fatigue. Brenda did not have a history of depression, but her new symptoms were beginning to weigh heavily on her mood. After her third glutathione IV, Brenda noted improvements. She felt steadier with walking, experienced fewer tremors, her energy improved and her friends commented she had a nice glow to her skin. She also felt more positive. She didn't realize that her physical health had started to affect her mental health. Now she wanted to do more for herself.

Prior to the changes with glutathione, Brenda resigned herself to thinking her slow decline in health was just a result of her age. She was 49 and many of her friends were on several prescriptions. Brenda realized she had more control over this decline than she thought. It is wonderful to witness the drive and motivation we can have when we get a taste of feeling better.

Another IV worth noting is vitamin C. It can support collagen production, in addition to providing other general health benefits. Here are some of the reasons patients might choose these IVs:

- Increased collagen production
- Immune system support
- Supportive care during cancer treatment

Also popular among patients at our clinic are Phosphatidylcholine (PC) IV therapies. PC is another nutrient that can be taken orally as well as in IV form. PC is found in eggs, soybeans, sunflower and other foods. The brain uses PC to make acetylcholine, a key communicator between neurons. It is also used by our cells to create healthy, fluid membranes for moving nutrients in and toxins out. If you suffer from rashes like eczema and hives, you likely have a fair amount of toxins built up in your tissues and would benefit from PC.

We offer PC in the IV form to support detoxification. Our bodies are like big fish - we bioaccumulate toxins we are exposed to over our lifetime. Some of us are better than others at neutralizing and removing these toxins, meaning we bioaccumulate less. Have you had a job where you were exposed to multiple chemicals? Maybe you grew up in a home with lead paint or an industrial building two streets down? We were all exposed to leaded gas until the mid-90's.

In today's world, it is basically impossible to steer clear of toxins. You may think of living in the countryside as better, but even this can lead to heavy pesticide exposure from nearby farms. PC IVs and oral therapies allow us to address this toxicity. PC research shows that it cleans up our cell membranes so we can get things in and out of our cells more efficiently. When we clean up chemicals that we are exposed to, our metabolism improves. We see skin clearing up and energy improves as well. PC has been used in Europe since 2002 to break down fat cells.

There are many additional nutrients that can be added to your IV schedule when appropriate. We will always discuss the reasons for our recommendations. The research articles addressing IV nutrients are abundant. There are B vitamins that benefit skin and detoxification, trace minerals that help with hair growth, and nutrients that are vital for energy and wound healing. IV therapies are not an alternative to cosmetic injections, but they can enhance the benefits of the injection procedures.

CHAPTER 6

Should I Try
That Face Cream?

E very health store, department store and even your neighborhood grocery have luxury skin creams advertised as the next best thing. We see the words "skin-firming" and "anti-aging" everywhere we look, but do these products really give you the changes you want? Even men have a long list of skin products to try, sometimes for acne, sometimes for hair growth. It's difficult looking at these choices and knowing which is best. It's even harder to figure out what else they are giving you, if not firmer skin. Heavy metals? Chemicals like parabens? Possibly.

Melissa, a patient of ours for several years, already struggled with sensitive skin. Recently, we discovered that chemicals in her new hypoallergenic facial serum were creating a problem. Usually she could avoid irritation by looking for a few known triggers, namely something called propylene glycol (PG). Any product with PG created an itchy red rash that lasted up to a week. Melissa was excited when she started a new anti-wrinkle serum free of PG and didn't see any trace of rash. Roughly six weeks into using the serum, Melissa was in our office complaining of hives and daily sinus congestion. There were not a lot of hives, but they popped up at least 5 times each week and she could not see a pattern. Sometimes they were on her forehead and neck, but other times on her forearms and legs. Having many allergies, it was not unusual for her to get the occasional itchy hive, or to have a stuffy nose. Since her diet and supplements had not changed and she didn't take any prescription medications, we discussed her current soaps and body products. The facial serum seemed like the most likely cause based on timing, so we decided she should take a break from it. Sure enough, after removing that product from daily use, her hives were gone a week later and so was her congestion.

Is it unusual to see a facial product affect other areas of the body, such as hives on a leg or a stuffy nose? Surprisingly, we see it often. Our skin absorbs much of what we put on it, meaning the whole body can potentially react if it sees a toxin or allergen. Melissa's product, though listed as "hypo-allergenic," contained 37 ingredients. Some of those ingredients were even ones regarded as toxic by much of the health industry, such as parabens. We had no way of knowing whether she was sensitive to one of those parabens, the yellow dye or any of the other 35 ingredients. What we *did* know was that we could decrease her risk of reactions by choosing more natural alternatives that contained fewer ingredients. Not everyone's body gives a clear warning signal when exposed to low levels of toxins. That doesn't mean these chemicals are less toxic or less likely to build up in their tissues. Each and every one of us, regardless of symptoms, can benefit from fewer chemical exposures.

We introduced Melissa to a resource that we should all be using in our day-to-day lives: The Environmental Working Group. The EWG, for short, is a nonprofit research group that provides up-to-date information on everything from the safest fish, to which hand cream is least toxic. Their Skin Deep site is a vast database that provides specifics on different cosmetic products and rates them for safety.

Next, we agreed upon a new approach to reducing wrinkles for Melissa: A personalized topical treatment that included her own platelet rich plasma. This is something we create for patients to use on wrinkles after they have our anti-aging cosmetic injections, but it can be helpful for reducing fine lines even without injection therapies. We extracted her platelets after a blood draw and added them to an ozone-rich oil. She applied the oil to her face and neck every night and then used something called a derma roller. Micro-needling with the roller helps introduce the platelets and the ozone into the upper layer of skin where they can stimulate collagen production. As expected with so few ingredients, Melissa didn't experience any negative side effects, but she did notice firmer looking skin by the time we saw her eight weeks later.

If you've never heard of ozonated oils, you are not alone. You won't find ozonated oils on most beauty store shelves or in your local drug store, but you should. The oil is saturated with both ozone and oxygen molecules which are absorbed by your skin cells. Cellular oxygenation is important for healthy tissue regeneration and growth. This is why ozonated oils are gaining so much popularity in cosmetics. Topical ozone can even speed up tissue healing. More often, though, these oils are used for their antimicrobial benefits. In fact, they are well researched for exactly this. We use ozonated oils for fungal, bacterial and viral skin infections. Many common types of fungus, including those that cause ringworm and yeast rashes, are treatable with ozonated oil [11]. We've seen shingles, warts and cold sores, all viral, improve with daily use of these oils [12] and heal faster.

Debbie also became a fan of ozone oil, though not at first. Ozone and ozonated oils have a very distinct smell. Some people describe it as "fresh," but Debbie was not one of those people. For her the smell was unpleasant, but she was able to tolerate it in her cosmetic facial serum because she liked how much smoother and fuller her skin appeared. When she noticed athlete's foot returning, rather than pick up a tube of Lamisil like she'd used in the past, she tried the ozone oil. Debbie told us the rash was gone in 4 days, which was at least a week faster than she was used to.

One of our other longtime patients, Jenna, developed multiple cold sores during the start of her divorce. Stress usually triggers the viral sores for her, but this was worse than usual. Her over-the-counter products weren't working, and neither was the lysine and licorice topical she usually relied upon. Within 2 days of putting ozonated olive oil on them, all three lesions began to heal. Within a week, they were gone. She also noticed the oil helped her acne lesions, making them less red and inflamed. We make sure to introduce all our patients to the potential benefits of ozonated oils, whether it's to treat acne, a new infection, or help with general skin regeneration.

Another product our patients love is a compounded prescription face cream specifically designed to further reduce wrinkles and reverse thinning skin. This is popular after our PRP facial injections to help maintain the collagen growth and improved appearance of the skin. Compounded creams let us select non-toxic ingredients and personalize dosing to fit each patient's needs. We often combine bio-identical hormones with strong antioxidants such as vitamin C.

CHAPTER 7

My Hair Needs A Makeover, Too

Debbie's main frustration was her aging skin. Once she was making headway on this, she decided she wanted to figure out why her hair was thinning. She noticed that it seemed to be falling out less with the treatments she was doing now. She also realized stress was a piece of the puzzle, especially work stress.

Hair loss is often connected with decreased circulation and nutrient deficiencies. There are genetic factors at play as well, and chronic health conditions that can all affect our hair. Dihydrotestosterone DHT levels (a result of testosterone conversion) can be normal in a blood test but elevated in the scalp, which contributes to hair loss. We offer a unique combination of treatments to improve hair loss, depending on the cause. Research has shown that red light therapy can significantly help with androgenic (male pattern baldness) and other types of hair loss in both men and women. It is a safe, relaxing treatment that stimulates hair growth when used a few times per week. This is what Debbie opted for.

Within two weeks, Debbie's hair loss slowed significantly. It used to be all over her hands in the shower and on the bathroom floor after drying her hair. Now she was only noticing a few hairs in her hands or on the floor. This added to her already growing confidence.

Another treatment that can be helpful is using a handheld tool with very small needles to apply your own platelets to your scalp. We perform a blood draw, separate out your platelets and add them to a personalized serum. This is kept in the refrigerator. A few nights a week, you can apply this in the convenience of your own home. Over time, you will start to see improvement. The serum is made monthly. Despite the needles, this does not hurt.

Scalp injections are the other treatment option we use for thinning hair. Your platelets are prepared similarly to the PRP for facial injections. Again, very small needles are used and it is virtually painless. Wearing a hat for the rest of the day covers any indication that you had work performed. Aside from a few small needle marks that show up after the treatment, there is no recovery time needed. You can also add the home platelet application to this treatment for even better results. It takes time for your hair cycle to show the results, but you will see them and so will others.

Greg was thrilled when he saw himself in his 30 year high school reunion photos. He was one of the only ones with a full head of hair. No one knew that a year ago he was suffering from hair thinning and a receding hairline before getting PRP injections. Prior to the procedure, he felt that his thinner hair made him look a lot older and was depleting his confidence. Now he continues to come in for the light therapy to keep his scalp and hair healthy. He also returns for injections once per year.

Like anything in health care and with the human body, these treatments work better when we look at the whole picture. If Debbie didn't get a handle on her stress, she wouldn't have the time to make her health and appearance a priority. We are always more successful when we have balance in our lives. Pretend your health is a 4-legged chair. One leg is your physical health, one is your emotional health, one is financial health and one is social health. What happens when 1-2 of these are missing or not secure?

In the next chapters, we will discuss how to get the most out of your investment. The injections and topicals are important, however so are the lifestyles you lead and the foods that you eat. You have the ability to improve your skin and hair starting today.

CHAPTER 8

Feed Your Skin The Foods It Deserves

When it comes to skin health, you can support yourself through diet, or you can fuel inflammation and aging. This may sound like an exaggeration, but it's not. The nutrients you absorb through your digestive tract are the building blocks for new skin cells, collagen, and hair. Nutritional deficiencies starve your cells of what they need to survive and divide. These same deficiencies hamper your ability to produce hormones, which contributes to the aging process. Even your immune system suffers when you are lacking certain vitamins and minerals, making your skin more susceptible to infections and rashes.

Sarah, a patient with a chronic digestive disorder known as Crohn's Disease, is a great example of how nutritional deficiencies wreak havoc on skin and hair. When we first saw Sarah, the main focus was reducing her abdominal pain and inflammation. As her digestive symptoms became better controlled, we had the chance to spend more time focusing on her skin concerns. Mostly she felt upset by a common rash called keratosis pilaris, which creates hard bumps on your arms and legs. She also felt like she was looking too old for her age, which was only 43. The prior year was a tough one, involving a "flare" in her gut symptoms. When the digestive tract is inflamed, the ability to absorb suffers. Sarah couldn't get enough out of the food she did eat, and she couldn't eat as much food as she needed. Even after the flare resolved, her skin showed signs of stress.

We decided PRP facial injections would help with the lines around her eyes and forehead, but first we needed to build her system back up. Stimulating collagen growth in her face wouldn't be nearly as effective if her body didn't have the right nutrients to support that tissue. In Sarah's case, we decided to focus on a combination of intravenous and oral vitamins and minerals, an individualized diet plan that wouldn't aggravate her condition, and daily collagen peptides. Within 4 weeks Sarah's skin appeared fuller and firmer, simply from the nutritional support. She even noticed her hair seemed fuller. When the little red bumps on her arms and legs didn't improve, we altered her diet to add more fatty acids and started supplementing vitamin A. It took another month, but we were all pleased to see the bumps receding. We started the cosmetic injections to further decrease wrinkles in the second month of treatment.

Sarah's experience is a good example because it demonstrates the importance of an individualized plan. PRP facial injections work similarly on all of us by stimulating collagen production. But what if something gets in the way of that new collagen? In Sarah's case, that *something* was going to be nutritional deficiencies. Her diet was key in her healing process and her skin's health.

Overabundance of unhealthy, pro-inflammatory foods is just as damaging to skin as nutritional deficiencies. We bet you've never heard anyone exclaim "Wow, my skin looks so great after I eat that pizza!" A diet full of sugar, processed grains and poor quality fats contributes to inflammation and hormone imbalances. If you are one of the lucky ones, you might only notice a bit of oily skin or puffy eyes the morning after a junk food binge. For most of us, it's also followed by a bout of acne, eczema or other inflammatory rash. Sometimes you don't even know how good your skin can look until you remove these things for a few weeks.

Debbie liked to describe her face as "rosy," and the occasional pimple and small red veins on her cheeks pointed toward rosacea. Her rash was mild and since her diet had room for change, we didn't prescribe medication. Debbie's diet wasn't horrible by most standards, and she never ate fast food. However, she did eat a lot of simple carbohydrates and vegetable oil. Breakfast was usually whole grain toast with I Can't Believe It's Not Butter! and coffee. She preferred salads for lunch and homemade dinners with chicken, bread and a vegetable. Snacks were usually pretzels or pita chips, a cheese stick, or chocolate covered raisins. These foods increase insulin levels (we all need this hormone, but too much is inflammatory!) and omega 6 fatty acids, which we discuss below. The first thing Debbie did was start a plan that removed the grain-based snacks and added in more proteins and better fats. This included wild fish, grass fed beef, nuts and seeds. We educated her about healthier dietary fats, and she began using avocado and olive oil. After 1 week, Debbie noticed she didn't have any more pimples on her cheeks, the redness was almost entirely gone, and she lost 3 pounds. She missed her comfort foods, but said the change was worth it.

One of the reasons too much bad food ages your skin is the production of advanced glycation end products (AGEs). These unpleasant proteins and fats are a source of inflammation, found in many processed foods, which add to overall oxidative stress. Too much oxidation slows your ability to heal and generate new cells, including your skin. AGEs are the same offenders that contribute to heart disease and other chronic diseases. While it is impossible to avoid all AGEs, we can limit animal products such as dairy and meat which contain higher amounts.

Since cooking at a high temperature quickly increases AGEs, imagine how much oxidative stress and inflammation your body faces from a deep fried meal [13]. We provide our patients with nutrition guidelines and meal examples to help minimize exposure to AGEs.

You've probably been told at some point to start taking fish oil. Maybe you are taking it right now. One of the reasons fish oil and other essential fatty acid supplements are beneficial is because most of us have an imbalance of omega 3 and omega 6 fatty acids. Fish oils provide extra omega 3, which we take to balance out our excess intake of omega 6. Could you have a deficiency in omega 3 fatty acids? It's possible. Are you eating an excessive amount of omega 6 fatty acids? Almost certainly.

The average American diet is overrun with omega 6 fatty acids, some of which directly increase your own production of inflammatory fats and proteins. Omega 3 fatty acids have anti-inflammatory effects, so you can imagine how important it is to balance these. If we lived on fresh fish, fruits and vegetables, our ratio would be balanced. Instead, the modern Western world consumes primarily those foods highest in omega 6: vegetable oils, grains, and meat from animals raised on those same grains. Even "health foods" like peanut butter contribute to this imbalance. Peanut butter is higher in arachidonic acid, which is more inflammatory than nut butters such as almond or cashew. Excess of certain nutrients is just as bad for body and skin as too little.

With so many potential nutritional deficiencies and excesses, where do we start? In our practice, we establish the foundation for healthy skin with a healthy, personalized diet plan. If there are known nutritional deficiencies, such as iron-deficiency anemia, supplementation is included. If we suspect a hidden deficiency such as biotin or vitamin B12, we may rely on a blood test so that we target the correct nutrients. The diet plan is not extreme, but it does require you to make changes to your daily habits and food choices.

Though each diet plan is adjusted to meet personal nutritional and lifestyle needs, they all emphasize three key principles. The plans are 1) anti-inflammatory, 2) lower in anti-nutrients such as lectins, and 3) centered around whole foods. When we switch to a diet comprised of whole foods, it automatically removes the processed options such as breads, sweets and junk food we all know are bad for us. It's not hard to make these changes, but our patients appreciate a clear guide on what to eat and what to avoid.

There are some obvious foods like sugar that are inflammatory for everyone, and best removed. Sugar often hides in condiments and even health foods such as yogurt. Other potentially inflammatory foods like nightshade family produce (peppers, tomatoes, potatoes, etc.) won't be restricted unless you are sensitive to them. An anti-inflammatory diet works best when we identify your unique sensitivities, both through symptoms and through a blood test. Lectins, phytic acids and other "anti-nutrients" are also reduced via our diet plans. These are naturally occurring in most foods, but at high levels they bind important nutrients and can interfere with your ability to absorb the vitamins and minerals you need. Anti-nutrients are also difficult for the digestive tract to break down, which means they can add to irritation and inflammation in the gut. Grains and nuts are a common source of these. We see the best changes in skin when we adjust how much of these you eat, and how you prepare them before meal time.

When we need to target a nutritional deficiency, the quickest and most powerful treatment is intravenous (IV) therapy. An IV with B vitamins or vitamin C will immediately boost blood levels without digestion getting in the way. Sometimes healing the digestive tract and increasing nutrient absorption from food and supplements takes time. IV therapies allow patients to feel better and see results right away. Intramuscular injections work well for certain nutrients, and they also bypass concerns about absorption in the gut. For our patients with healthy, happy bellies, we can focus on replenishing specific nutrients through a combination of dietary adjustments and supplements. Not all vitamins are equal, and often we find it necessary to prescribe activated vitamins or liposomal forms to further enhance absorption. It's extremely important that any supplement you take be high quality. We only prescribe vitamins, minerals and other micronutrients that have undergone vigorous quality testing to ensure they contain what they state on their labels.

The most common nutritional deficiencies we see in patients with skin complaints include vitamin C, biotin, vitamin A, iron and protein. Remember Sarah? One of the IV therapies she found most helpful was vitamin C. Though she was mostly concerned about the keratosis pilaris rash and her wrinkles, we noted a pattern of dry skin, slow-healing scratches and gums that bled easily. Sarah needed vitamin C, and she needed it fast. We started with three IVs, then switched to liposomal (oral) vitamin C for her to use at home.

We find patients experience the greatest results when they make changes to their diets and daily routines. This is key to creating healthier skin and optimizing long-term health and wellness. In the next chapter, we will discuss additional ways that you can support skin and whole body health through detoxification. Many of these steps can be taken at home before, during and after your cosmetic procedures.

CHAPTER 9

Detox Your Face

Detoxification products, diet plans, shakes and supplements are everywhere. It's impossible to pick up a health magazine without seeing some mention of detoxification. Are these plans worthwhile? Are they necessary? We will tell you what we tell all our patients: detox support can be helpful, but it needs to be done the right way.

The body is a master at detoxification. Every cell in your body is designed to mobilize, process and expel toxins that are then filtered out of your system via gut, kidneys, liver, skin and lungs. A beneficial detox plan is one that enhances your body's own detox pathways while decreasing the number of toxins you are exposed to. If a plan involves a cabinet full of cleansing products, it's probably creating more work for your liver rather than helping you.

Think of your body as a factory. New materials are constantly being brought in and processed to create a product. This work simultaneously creates garbage or things that need to be recycled. Imagine your cells have 100 employees doing this work, just enough to keep everything running smoothly. Your body is doing this every moment of every day. The food you eat, the water you drink, and the air you breathe are being used by your cells to make very important products: energy, new cells, hormones and more. Meanwhile, different employees in your cells and major organs are gathering up and removing the garbage. To keep it simple, this is what we call "detox."

If your factory creates too much garbage at once, or someone drops off a bunch of their own garbage, your employees struggle and the trash builds up. Sadly, this is the state that many of us live in. Our cells do their best to remove the toxins we create and acquire, but we are continually being saturated with chemical food additives, pesticides, prescription medications, and heavy metals. These create more work for your system, which slows down your ability to detox.

Now let's say you are making the same amount of garbage, but a third of your staff call in sick. Suddenly, you have the same problem. Waste products build up, and the only way to keep up is to get more employees on the job. A lot of things might cause you to have fewer employees. Nutrient deficiencies are a common cause of this, but so are dehydration and lack of sleep. For some people, genetics lead to a smaller staff.

Are detoxification and skin connected? Of course. Skin, after all, is one of your major detox organs. Waste products, your body's "garbage," are excreted in your perspiration from sweat glands on a daily basis. You can even think of skin as one of your factory's primary employees. But what about general appearance and health of your skin? How does detoxification improve that? Most of our patients report that their skin has less acne and fewer rashes after we've started detoxification protocols. It may sound cliché, but we usually hear "My skin is brighter!" A majority of the benefits these patients see is probably due to better hormone balance and lower inflammation as a result of fewer toxins in the body. When the liver has fewer environmental toxins to battle, it is better at keeping up with processing the hormones and other metabolites you already produce every day.

Even something as simple as drinking more water can improve your skin. Unless you have a medical condition that requires you to limit fluids, we recommend increasing your water intake to at least half your body weight in ounces. You will see the difference within just a few days. This was something Debbie figured out a while before coming to our clinic. She'd read once that drinking more water helped with weight loss. After increasing to 120 ounces every day, she didn't see the rapid fat loss she'd hoped for, but her skin was less dry, wrinkles less prominent and her eyes were less puffy.

Although we don't require a detox protocol as part of our program for natural cosmetic injections, we do offer it when appropriate. The anti-inflammatory diet plan does a lot already, simply by decreasing exposures to food additives and pesticides. Remember, your body's ability to detox is very sensitive to how many toxins it is exposed to minute by minute. Don't underestimate the power of removing chemical-laden foods, decreasing medications when appropriate and limiting environmental exposures. Bio-accumulation affects every one of us.

Sometimes stronger detoxification support is necessary, and when it is, we make it a priority. One patient, Lindsey, came to us with fatigue, body pain, sinus congestion and 4 months of hair loss after exposure to toxic black mold in her apartment. Even after she moved out, leaving furniture and personal belongings behind, she was still losing hair one month later. Stachybotrys, the black mold she encountered, produces mycotoxins that can accumulate in the blood and lymph during large exposures. In her case, the sinus congestion stopped right away, but her achy joints and hair loss didn't begin to improve until we treated her with IV glutathione and supplements that helped bind and remove the mycotoxins. By 6 weeks into treatments, she reported feeling 80% back to normal. Her hair hadn't yet started to grow back in, but she was no longer losing it rapidly.

For most patients, we keep it simple when recommending detox support. In addition to cleaner food choices and hydration, we educate about options such as intermittent fasting and ways to increase sweating. Intermittent fasting for 12-18 hours can be done daily or a few days per week. It gives the body, especially the liver, a chance to work unhindered by incoming foods. Intermittent fasting can also help to stabilize blood sugar fluctuations by making you more sensitive to your own insulin.

Exercise is one of the best ways to stimulate metabolism in your cells and promote sweating, both of which increase detoxification. It also helps to stimulate the bowels, which are responsible for helping you to remove waste products every day. When exercise capacity is limited due to injury or another disability, we recommend infrared sauna. Exercise and sauna therapy may sound very basic, but a healthy body is capable of doing its own detox when we can reduce toxin exposures and support basic detoxification pathways.

Another popular form of detox support is colon hydrotherapy. Since many of your daily toxins are excreted by way of the colon, cleansing the colon itself aids in detoxification. This is best performed by a licensed therapist who gently infuses your colon with water. We recommend choosing a therapist who is board certified in colonics by the International Association for Colon Hydrotherapy (I-ACT). For certified therapists in your region, visit www.i-act.org.

Remember, it is easy to get overwhelmed by health fads. We are constantly bombarded with information. During this program, we want you to learn things that will help you and those you care about be as healthy as possible. We added a list of resources at the end of this book so you will have a reference guide as well. We also continually update our website and Facebook page with tools that we see work.

CHAPTER 10

Isn't There A Test For That?

The natural aging process of our skin proceeds even when we are in a state of perfect health. Your basic blood work will likely be within range, and even your hormones might be normal for your age. Knowing this, is it worth running other blood tests? Which tests are worth your time and money? You may see advertisements with information about testing that can improve your health. What is out there and what works? We will make this clear for you and provide you with testing that is individualized to meet your needs.

We require basic blood chemistries before we can start injections and IVs, but there are two main reasons we might request additional labs. First, to rule out specific deficiencies or conditions based on your general health symptoms. Second, to provide us with information so we can optimize your health and your skin. Most often, these additional labs are optional. Your symptoms or your desire to optimize results directs us toward which tests are appropriate. There are several categories of tests that we will discuss.

Sometimes symptoms of a deficiency are very clear, and a major contributor to your skin and hair concerns. Stephanie was one such case. She scheduled as a new patient for PRP scalp injections to address thinning hair. During the intake, she mentioned fatigue and at least one year of very heavy periods since starting perimenopause. Hair loss, fatigue, and heavy bleeding combined to paint a picture of iron deficiency. Her basic labs didn't show anemia yet, but when we ran her iron levels, they were extremely low. Stephanie worked with her gynecologist to slow the bleeding and we started her on daily iron. The PRP scalp injections helped to speed up hair regrowth, and treating iron deficiency prevented further hair loss. If we proceeded with the injections before identifying and treating the deficiency, Stephanie would not have seen good results.

When Debbie scheduled for her PRP facial injections, she was primarily concerned with her wrinkles and "sagging" skin. As we discussed in prior chapters, she did have a bit of fatigue and some achy joints, but she always assumed it was normal for a woman her age. Even her menopausal symptoms weren't horrible, but she did have hot flashes a few days per week. She'd had food allergies in her 40s, but didn't have any of the digestive symptoms that once troubled her. Despite feeling generally good, Debbie wanted the best possible outcome from her cosmetic treatments and suspected hormones and certain foods might not be helping her skin.

We ordered blood work to check hormone levels and look for food intolerances. Debbie had low estrogen, which we expected, but she also had very low testosterone. When low, these hormone levels contribute to the progression of wrinkles and thinning skin. They can also contribute to lower energy and hot flashes. After more discussion and a deeper look at her menopausal symptoms, we prescribed a low dose of bio-identical hormones. The hot flashes were gone within the first week and the skin on her face, hands and legs was less dry.

Debbie's food panel showed high antibodies to gluten and eggs which she ate every day. Even when we remove inflammatory foods like sugar, other healthy options such as eggs might be triggering inflammation depending on a person's immune system. Knowing what Debbie reacted to made it easier to create an anti-inflammatory diet plan for her.

Let's discuss the tests we've found most helpful in our clinic, starting with basic screening labs. These labs are often ordered by primary care physicians during your annual physical exam. They include a chemistry panel, blood cell panel, and basic thyroid tests. Additional standard labs we may request include an iron panel, vitamin B12 and vitamin D. These give us an idea of how healthy your major organs are, whether you are anemic, and whether you are struggling with thyroid disease. If looked at very closely, they can also indicate borderline deficiencies in specific vitamins and minerals. Reference ranges for labs are based on averages, not optimal levels. Physicians may interpret them in the different ways. A "normal" level is not always an optimal level.

Hormone panels - like the one ordered for Debbie - may be useful when we are hoping to optimize health, or when there are symptoms that suggest a hormone imbalance. For hair loss in women, high testosterone levels might be the cause. Also, high testosterone and other steroid hormones can cause acne. Hormone imbalance can contribute to acne rosacea as well, and of course, hormone deficiencies early in life will speed up skin aging. Weight gain around the face and neck, both in men and women, can be linked to hormone changes. Metabolism is sensitive to our gender hormones, just like skin. When men come into our clinic with early balding, we need to take testosterone levels into consideration. If they are quickly converting testosterone to the potent dihydrotestosterone (DHT), they are likely to see continued hair loss unless the converting enzyme is treated.

Thyroid and cortisol hormones are just as important as the gender hormones. Our clinic sees deficiencies of both hormones more often than we see high levels. Imbalances in either direction can cause skin and hair changes. A basic TSH thyroid screening is commonly run by primary care physicians, but thyroid disorders can be easily missed with this test. If we have high suspicion of thyroid dysfunction, we will order more extensive thyroid labs. Common symptoms associated with thyroid disorders include hair loss, dry skin, weight and energy fluctuations. Low cortisol, one of the hormones that helps you deal with stress, can cause hair loss as well. We also see more inflammatory rashes like eczema in patients with low cortisol.

Sometimes genetic testing is helpful in understanding persistent and displeasing changes in skin and hair. Marie came to our clinic upset about ten years of slowly thinning hair. Her genetic screening revealed a defect in the enzyme responsible for utilizing biotin, a vitamin that is essential for healthy hair growth. Another patient's genetic screening revealed a decreased ability to activate beta carotene, the lovely antioxidant that makes carrots orange, into active vitamin A. This was significant in her skin health because she also had keratosis pilaris that can result from a vitamin A deficiency. We cannot alter your genetics, but sometimes knowing about specific defects allows us to target nutritional or hormonal imbalances caused by them.

If you've noticed that what goes into your mouth shows up on your skin, you are not imagining it. Gut health is a major factor in overall inflammation as discussed in previous chapters. Our patients often see inflammatory rashes like acne, rosacea and eczema improve with dietary changes. Dark circles and swelling under the eyes also respond to identifying and removing problem foods. When we are not sure which foods might be contributing, we run a blood test to measure antibodies for food intolerances. This provides a targeted list of foods to reduce or remove from your diet, versus starting a broad and time-consuming elimination diet. Sometimes a stool panel will be recommended. Certain bacterial and parasitic infections in the digestive tract cause nutrient deficiencies and rashes. A comprehensive stool panel looks at whether you have an abundance of good versus bad bacteria, hidden parasitic infections, low digestive enzymes and even checks for inflammation.

While a simple iron panel or vitamin B12 level is sufficient for most patients, sometimes we recommend an extensive micronutrient panel to looks at various vitamins, minerals and antioxidants. This allows us to catch underlying causes for skin and hair changes that might otherwise be missed. One easily missed deficiency is biotin. Low levels of biotin are not common, but when they occur they can cause substantial hair loss. Women breastfeeding for many years may be low in biotin, and those struggling with poor digestion may be at risk. Even something as obscure as eating raw egg whites for fitness training can cause a biotin deficiency. Gathering information about antioxidant levels can also be helpful. If someone is deficient in these it may suggest a high level of inflammation depleting their antioxidants, or a nutrient deficiency. Either way, low antioxidant levels impair the body's ability to defend against oxidative damage that contributes to skin aging.

Testing for heavy metal toxicity is another option for patients with hair loss, usually when there is a known exposure or other suspicious health complaints. Symptoms of heavy metal toxicity tend to be vague and hard to identify, such as impaired immune function, poor memory, fatigue and more. We take the whole picture into consideration, including job and home exposures. Each of us is exposed to metals daily via car exhaust, foods, water and other environmental exposures. However, certain lifestyle factors increase the risk for exposure and bio-accumulation of heavy metals. If heavy metals are present at high levels in the tissues, they can be reduced through chelation therapies. The negative impact of heavy metal toxicity on hair growth is well researched [14].

We recommend new patients bring copies of their most recent blood work whenever able. This sometimes reduces the need for additional labs. It also gives us an opportunity to learn more about your general health and potential contributors to skin and hair changes.

CHAPTER 11

Medical Myth Busters & Your Skin

We often overhear our patients discussing expert advice they came across via media. Sometimes it comes up because the advice seemed questionable to them, but they assumed it must be true. Who are these experts and where is this information coming from? Did our patients hear a physician on the radio or see them on TV? What is their training? Was it a post from "Facebook university" or an "expert" on nutrition who has zero training? Public figures often build a following without real training. When is the last time you stopped to check the credentials of an expert you came across online?

There's a lot of quality, reliable health information circulating in the media. For every good report, though, there seems to be 2-3 false claims. Many of these impact how people think about their skin and their overall health.

Here are some of our favorite health claims that often find their way into our clinic. We hope this helps to further your understanding of your body, and how to keep your skin glowing. Real change is possible, but it's important not to fall for false claims.

The baggy, loose skin under your eyes is just age.

You hear that there is nothing you can do. You are aging. Those under-eye bags are all in your genes. Take some Ambien to sleep better or wear a better brand of concealer. You may have been told at make-up counters in the mall that it is from the way you are applying your make-up.

We want you to know, it's often more than just genetics and aging. Here's what you can do:

1. Have *reactions to foods tested*. Avoiding food intolerances can drastically change what you look like in photos. Have you noticed that week-to-week you can look different? Bloating and facial swelling can change in a matter of days. Anything that increases inflammation and fluid retention takes a toll. We

have seen patients who lose 5-8 pounds in a week just by removing foods intolerances from their diet. We like to test for a combination of antibodies via blood. Remember, not all tests are created equal and traditional allergy tests do not identify intolerances.

2. Improve your *sleep hygiene* before you try a pill. Turn off the Wi-Fi in your house before bed. Unplug all electronics when you can. Turn your cell phone to airplane mode. There is plenty of research to support this. Darken your bedroom. You should make your bedroom be as if you were camping: Pitch dark until the sun comes up. Zero electronics. Use battery alarm clocks or your phone on airplane mode as an alarm clock. There is a wonderful website full of useful information and research in our resource section. Also, no caffeine after noon. It does affect your sleep. Limit the caffeine you have in the morning. Look into buying blue light blocking glasses and wearing them before bed. You may look silly, but they work when used consistently.

3. *Hydrate!* It is helpful to start drinking clean water and drink more of it. Buy a filter for your house. We have some links on our website. Stop drinking out of plastic bottles. The chemicals from the plastics have hormone-like effects. If you are on a diuretic, or have a health condition that needs monitoring, consult

with your physician before dramatically changing water intake. However, for the average person, a simple trick is to divide your weight by half and drink that much in ounces each day. In other words, if you weigh 120 pounds, shoot for at least 60 ounces. You will notice that you have more energy during the day and crave less coffee, sugar and carbs. We find it helpful to use rubber bands to remember your daily tally. Buy a glass or stainless steel liter bottle and place 2 rubber bands at the top. If you are aiming for 60 ounces, every time your finish your bottle, move a rubber band to the bottom. You are done when all the rubber bands are at the bottom.

4. Try not to smash one side of your face into your pillow at night. Have you noticed that your lines are not symmetrical? This can often be due to how you sleep.

Your acne has nothing to do with what you eat.

Trust us, you don't have a deficiency in Accutane or antibiotics. Repeated courses of antibiotics are harmful to your digestive health and immune system. They wreak havoc on our mitochondria, the little powerhouses that energize cells. We develop resistant strains of bacteria when we use them too often. Our patients are repeatedly told by doctors that what they eat does not affect their skin. If you've ever had acne and tried different diets, you already know this is false.

Here's what you can do to decrease acne breakouts:

1. Have *reactions to foods tested*. See above. This is almost always a piece of the puzzle.
2. Manage your *stress*. Big fluctuations in stress hormones alter oil production in the skin, which can worsen acne. Where is the stress coming from? Figure out ways to minimize it.
3. Support your digestive health by *minimizing refined grains, sugar, and alcohol*. Most of your immune system lives in your gut, so a little inflammation in your belly will affect your entire body. Try very hard to *avoid GMOs*. Common sources are corn, soy, and packaged foods.
4. Calendar your breakouts. Are they connected to your cycle? If so, we focus on improving your *hormone balance*.

Rosacea just happens with age, **but an antibiotic is all you need**.

Sound familiar? Like acne, you are handed an antibiotic ointment or pill. And like acne, inflammation is taking a toll and showing up on your face. The antibiotic may help reduce the appearance, but what about the underlying inflammation?

Here's what you can do to decrease rosacea:

1. Have *reactions to foods tested*. See above.
2. *Hormone testing*. Balancing your hormones can drastically improve your skin. Rosacea tends to increase in women around menopausal age when there are large shifts in estrogen levels.
3. *Digestive testing*. If you don't have access to testing, simply start by cleaning up your diet as mentioned above. Add a teaspoon of organic apple cider vinegar to a small amount of water before meals. Improving your digestive enzyme levels can improve your digestive health and can lead to calmer, less inflamed skin.
4. *Topical Ozone Oil* also helps improve the color and texture of your skin. See our website for options.

Everyone gets thin hair when they reach a certain age.

Again, you will hear that you are just aging. Your thinning hair is nothing to worry about. Your basic labs are normal, so you are told it can't be iron or low thyroid. You will be told it is just genetics. You may even be told to take a pre-natal if you are female and still pre-menopausal. There is nothing unique about pre-natal vitamins except for extra folic acid, and furthermore, it's the inactive form. If women see improvements in hair growth before becoming pregnant, a basic multivitamin would have done the trick. If it's during pregnancy, the thickening hair is more likely due to the abundance of hormones.

Here's what you can do to improve your hair now:

1. *Hormone testing and balancing.* This may require low doses of bio-identical hormones, or it may be as simple as introducing herbal support and focused dietary changes. If you have symptoms of thyroid disease and your thyroid stimulating hormone (TSH) is within range, you might want to have your Free T3, Free T4, Reverse T3 and antibody levels tested.

2. *Nutrient testing* to rule out specific deficiencies known to cause hair loss, such as low biotin.

3. *Digestive testing.* Poor production of digestive enzymes can also contribute to hair loss if you aren't absorbing nutrients well.

4. *Topical Ozone Oil* applied with a derma roller can increase oxygen saturation of local tissues to feed hair roots and skin cells.

5. Work on minimizing *stress*. Acute stress, such as a motor vehicle accident or other trauma can cause sudden hair loss for 1-3 months.

6. Start a good quality *multi-vitamin and trace mineral supplement*. See our website for options.

The weight around your middle is due to high cortisol levels.

We hear this often. There are several ads on TV explaining how their company's supplement decreases cortisol and allows your belly fat to quickly melt away. Unless you have Cushing's Syndrome, chronic stress depletes cortisol levels over time. Cortisol-lowering herbs and nutrients won't magically slim your waist line or chin. There is no supplement that will work for spot reduction.

Here's what you can do to make changes now:

1. Have *reactions to food tested*. See above. This can drastically reduce bloating, including puffiness in your face, hands and feet.
2. Clean up your diet by *minimizing refined grains, sugar, and alcohol*. Start by decreasing your servings of grains to one per day, and remove cane sugar. Then you can continue to taper to grains no more than once a week. Decreasing sugar in your diet will make a massive change in your overall weight. After you've removed cane sugar, focus on other sources of excess sugar like juices and dried fruit. Don't forget hidden sources of

cane and other sugars, such as pasta sauces, yogurts, and alcoholic beverages. Within just a few days of a grain-free and sugar-free diet, you will start to have more energy and better moods.

3. Over time, losing body fat will result in both a leaner middle and a leaner jawline. Keep track of body fat percentage for more accurate monitoring.

I better wear sunscreen all of the time or I'll get skin cancer.

Yes, protecting yourself from harmful UV rays is important. However, not all sunscreens are equal in safety and effectiveness. Also, keep in mind that skin cancer rates are not higher if you live closer to the equator. If sun exposure alone increases your risk for skin cancer, shouldn't those rates be higher near the equator?

Here's what you should know about sunscreen:

1. Use appropriate forms of sunscreen with fewer *hormone-disruptive ingredients*. Zinc oxide and carrot seed oils are recommended. See links on our site.

2. Have your vitamin D tested. Having *adequate vitamin D* levels plays an important role in cancer prevention.

3. Whether or not you have a family history of skin cancer, *find a good dermatologist* to monitor your skin.

4. Also *consider tinting the windows of your vehicle* if you drive often. Have you noticed that one side of your face seems to have more sun damage?

We hope these health tips help you to feel motivated to create change in your life. We are in a time of information overload. It can be helpful to make small, consistent changes which after enough time become habits. The more you take control of your life, the more successful you will be. Let us do the work of filtering out quality health advice so that we can serve as a resource to you for concise, easy-to-follow treatment plans that will ensure your health success.

Also, keep in mind that nothing replaces daily self-care. When we surround ourselves with a healthy lifestyle and good habits, the results typically show on our face and entire body. Our patients see the best health changes when we can motivate them to create changes at home. As patients start to look and feel better, their vices fade. When you exercise more, you notice more energy and fewer cravings. Also, with health information that makes sense, motivation for change sticks.

In healthcare, and other parts of our lives, what works usually makes sense. Beware of advice that is not backed by research or a trained practitioner. Also, beware "one size fits all" recommendations. We see false claims every day that fit these patterns. Our program will give you safe, reliable results. It will happen - you will see.

CHAPTER 12

Conclusion

Now that you've made it to the end of the book, you probably have a better sense of how a natural cosmetic medicine program will benefit you and your skin. We are excited about this non-toxic, natural alternative to surgery and synthetic fillers, but more importantly, we are thrilled by the opportunity to help you make whole body health changes.

We wanted to introduce you to Debbie because she came in for younger looking skin, but left also *feeling* younger. In addition to leaving behind deep frown lines, Debbie discarded joint pain, fatigue, hot flashes, rosacea and the nagging insecurity that began plaguing her a few years ago. When Debbie last checked in with us, she was scheduling touch up injections 12 months from her last session and still feeling like a new person.

She kept the diet and lifestyle changes going, something she didn't feel motivated to do before starting the program.

Debbie's story is the perfect example of why we invest our passion and energy into therapies that promote the body's own regenerative capacity. Anti-aging medicine is about more than just stimulating new collagen in your face. It should encompass the whole body and support general wellness, whether through reducing inflammation or balancing hormones.

If you are still struggling with whether cosmetic injections are right for you, we hope that you've gained useful insight into other aspects of your health and daily life. While the program itself is focused on reducing wrinkles, firming skin and assisting hair growth, we want each of our patients to walk away with generalized health improvements. If you are low in biotin, every tissue in your body will benefit from supplementation, not just the thickness of your hair. Likewise, if your diet begins to change into one rich in omega 3 fatty acids and anti-inflammatory whole foods, you will notice changes in energy and your general wellbeing. You will also chip away at your risk for chronic diseases like diabetes, heart disease and cancer.

To help pull together everything you've just read, we will review the program in summary. We want you to feel familiar and comfortable with the process, including the importance of the procedures and lifestyle changes that are separate from the actual cosmetic injections.

Each new patient will meet with one of us for a full new patient intake so that we can get to know you, your health history, your concerns and needs. This includes a focused physical exam and a review of blood work. If labs are not available, we can order them for you on the day of your new patient visit. If we feel additional labs are indicated, they will be discussed and ordered with your permission. You will also leave with an outline of your personalized diet plan to begin right away. The new patient visit is an excellent time to ask us questions. We also look forward to hearing and understanding your goals and expectations.

After this new patient visit, you will already have a set of pre-scheduled appointments you made when you first signed up for the program. These include three cosmetic injection sessions, three Major Autohemotherapy IVs, and an additional follow up visit scheduled during the 3-month period. The IVs and injections can be done on back-to-back days or spread out depending on your scheduling and travel needs. For those traveling a significant distance, we can schedule over a 6-month period. If during the new patient visits we decide to add other supportive therapies, these will be added to your schedule. This might include an additional 1-3 Major Autohemotherapy IVs, a specific nutrient replenishing IV such as high dose vitamin C, or vitamin B injections. We will not recommend add-on procedures unless we feel they are indicated for you based on our intake and exam. It is important to us that you feel included and well-informed regarding this planning process. No changes will be made without your full consent.

There is a follow up office visit half-way through your three-month plan. We will evaluate and discuss visible changes in response to the therapies, and we will also focus on reviewing your progress with the diet. Have you noticed other changes than just those in your face? Are you feeling satisfied with the changes? There may be new labs to review, new questions and health concerns to address. We will also spend time discussing the topical regimen started at your first injection session, and your personalized home maintenance plan.

We look forward to seeing the increased self-confidence you develop by the end of this program. Our hope and our goal is to see it inspire you to continue investing time and energy into self-care. Your skin will thank you, and so will the rest of your body.

Citations

[1] de Aquino MS, Haddad A, Ferreira LM. *Assessment of quality of life in patients who underwent minimally invasive cosmetic procedures.* June.2013. URL: https://www.ncbi.nlm.nih.gov/pubmed/23519872

[2] Crinnion WJ. *Environmental medicine, part one: the human burden of environmental toxins and their common health effects.* Feb 2000. URL: https://www.ncbi.nlm.nih.gov/pubmed/10696119

[3] Alberts B, Johnson A, Lewish J, et al. *Epidermis and Its Renewal by Stem Cells.* 2002. URL:https://www.ncbi.nlm.nih.gov/books/NBK26865/

[4] Hillebrand GG, Liang Z, Yan X, Yoshii T. *New wrinkles on wrinkling: an 8-year longitudinal study on the progression of expression lines into persistent wrinkles.* Jun 2010. URL: https://www.ncbi.nlm.nih.gov/pubmed/20184587

[5] Raina D'souza, Ashwini Kini, Henston D'souza, Nitin Shetty, and Omkar Shetty. *Enhancing Facial Aesthetics with*

Muscle Retraining Exercises-A Review. Aug 2014. URL: https://www.ncbi.nlm.nih.gov/pmc/articles/PMC4190816/

[6] Alberts B, Johnson A, Lewis J, et al. *Fibroblasts and Their Transformations: The Connective-Tissue Cell Family.* 2002. URL: https://www.ncbi.nlm.nih.gov/books/NBK26889/

[7] Boyera N, Galey I, Bernard BA. *Effect of vitamin C and its derivatives on collagen synthesis and cross-linking by normal human fibroblasts.* June 1998. URL: https://www.ncbi.nlm.nih.gov/pubmed/18505499

[8] James Varani, Michael K. Dame, Laure Rittie, Suzanne E.G. Fligiel, Sewon Kang, Gary J. Fisher, and John J. Voorhees. *Decreased Collagen Production in Chronologically Aged Skin.* June 2006. URL: https://www.ncbi.nlm.nih.gov/pmc/articles/PMC1606623/

[9] Anson G, Kane MA, Lambros V. *Sleep Wrinkles: Facial Aging and Facial Distortion During Sleep.* Sep 2016. URL: https://www.ncbi.nlm.nih.gov/pubmed/27329660

[10] Manicourt DH, Druetz-Van Egeren A, Haazen L, Nagant de Deuxchaisnes C. Effects of tenoxicam and aspirin on the metabolism of proteoglycans and hyaluronan in normal and osteoarthritic human articular cartilage. Dec 1994. URL: https://www.ncbi.nlm.nih.gov/pubmed/7889262/

[11] Neveen S.I. Geweely. *Antifungal Activity of Ozonized Olive Oil (Oleozone).* URL: http://www.the-o-zone.cc/research/abstracts/002.pdf)

[12] Mattassi, R.M.D., D'Angelo F., M.D.M Franchina A., M.D., Bassi P., M.D. *Ozone as Therapy in Herpes Simplex and Herpes Zoster Diseases.* URL: http://www.the-o-zone.cc/research/abstracts/028.html

[13] J Am Diet Assoc. *Advanced Glycation End Products in Foods and a Practical Guide to Their Reduction in the Diet.* June 2010. URL: https://www.ncbi.nlm.nih.gov/pmc/articles/PMC3704564/

[14] Pierard GE. *Toxic effects of metals from the environment on hair growth and structure.* Aug 1979. URL: https://www.ncbi.nlm.nih.gov/pubmed/227944_

Resources

We have put together a list of some of our favorite websites, associations, and educators to help you have a place to look for more information. We continue to add research links to our website, www.lakeoswegohealth.com, weekly.

1. The American Academy of Ozontherapy: www.aaot.us
2. American College for Advancement in Medicine: www.acam.org
3. The Institute for Functional Medicine: www.functionalmedicine.org
4. Oregon Association of Naturopathic Physicians: www.oanp.org
5. The American Association of Naturopathic Physicians: www.naturopathic.org
6. Environmental Working Group: www.ewg.org
7. David Perlmutter MD: www.drperlmutter.com

8. Linus Pauling Institute: http://oregonstate.edu/ua/ncs/linus-pauling-institute
9. The International Academy of Oral Medicine & Toxicology: www.iaomt.org
10. The Weston A. Price Foundation®: www.westonaprice.org
11. Dr. Mercola: www.drmercola.com

Additional Research Articles

The following research articles are available online. Each contains information regarding skin and general health that we find beneficial.

Abuaf OK, Yildiz H, Baloglu H, and Bilgili ME, et al. *Histologic Evidence of New Collagen Formulation Using Platelet Rich Plasma in Skin Rejuvenation: A Prospective Controlled Clinical Study.* Dec 2016. URL:

https://www.ncbi.nlm.nih.gov/pubmed/27904271

Aguilar P, Hersant B, SidAhmed-Mezi M, Bosc R, Vidal L, Meningaud JP. *Novel technique of vulvo-vaginal rejuvenation by lipofilling and injection of combined platelet-rich-plasma and hyaluronic acid: a case-report.* Jul. 2016. URL:

https://www.ncbi.nlm.nih.gov/pubmed/27512643

Anitua E, Pino A, Jaen P, Orive G. *Plasma Rich in Growth Factors Enhances Wound Healing and Protects from Photo-oxidative Stress in Dermal Fibroblasts and 3D Skin Models.* 2016. URL:

https://www.ncbi.nlm.nih.gov/pubmed/26927211

Barcelos RC, Vey LT, and Segat HJ, et al. *Cross-generational trans fat intake exacerbates UV radiation-induced damage in rat skin.* Jul 2014. URL:

https://www.ncbi.nlm.nih.gov/pubmed/24694906

Berardi AC, Oliva F, and Berardocco M, et.al. *Thyroid hormones increase collagen I and cartilage oligomeric matrix protein (COMP) expression in vitro human tenocytes.* Nov 2014. URL :

https://www.ncbi.nlm.nih.gov/pubmed/25489544

Biesman BS, Bowe WP. *Effect of Midfacial Volume Augmentation With Non Animal Stabilized Hyaluronic Acid on the Nasolabial Fold and Global Aethestic Appearance.* Sep 2015. URL:

https://www.ncbi.nlm.nih.gov/pubmed/26355611

Cavallo C, Roffi A, and Grigolo B, et al. *Platelet-Rich Plasma: The Choice of Activation Method Affects the Release of Bioactive Molecules.* Sep 2016. URL:

https://www.ncbi.nlm.nih.gov/pubmed/27672658

de Aquino MS1, Haddad A, Ferreira LM. *Assessment of quality of life in patients who underwent minimally invasive cosmetic procedures.* June 2013. URL:

10.1007/s00266-012-9992-0

Dermatoendocrinol. Ruta Gancevicine, Aikaterini I. Liakou, and Athanasios Theodoridis, et. al. *Skin anti-aging strategies.* Jul 2012. URL:

https://www.ncbi.nlm.nih.gov/pmc/articles/
PMC3583892/#!po=0.239234

Elnehrawy NY, Ibrahim ZA1, Eltoukhy AM, Nagy HM. *Assessment of the efficacy and safety of single platelet-rich plasma injection on different types and grades of facial wrinkles.* Jul 2016. URL:

http://onlinelibrary.wiley.com/doi/10.1111/jocd.12258/abstract

El Taieb MAI, Ibrahim H, Nada EA, Seif Al-Din M. *Platelets rich plasma versus minoxidil 5% in treatment of alopecia areata: A trichoscopic evaluation.* Oct 2016. URL:

https://www.ncbi.nlm.nih.gov/pubmed/27791311

Giacomoni PU1, Declercq L, Hellemans L, Maes D. *Aging of human skin: review of a mechanistic model and first experimental data.* Apr. 2000. URL:

  https://www.ncbi.nlm.nih.gov/pubmed/10995026

Ivanov V, Ivanova S, and Kalinovsky T, et.al. *Inhibition of collagen synthesis by select calcium and sodium channel blockers can be mitigated by ascorbic acid and ascorbyl palmitate.* May 2016. URL:

  https://www.ncbi.nlm.nih.gov/pubmed/27335688

Ulusal MD, Betul Gozel. J Cosmet Dermatol. *Platelet-rich plasma and hyaluronic acid - an efficient biostimulation method for face rejuvenation.* Sep 2016. URL:

  http://onlinelibrary.wiley.com/doi/10.1111/jocd.12271/abstract

Keiko Asakura, Yuji Nishiwaki, and Ai Milojevic, et al. Lifestyle Factors and Visible Skin Aging in a Population of Japanese Elders. Sep 2009. URL:

  https://www.ncbi.nlm.nih.gov/pmc/articles/PMC3924128/

Miyata S. [*Supplementation of trace elements in the general medicine*]. Jul 2016. URL:

  https://www.ncbi.nlm.nih.gov/pubmed/27455795

Norval M1, Lucas RM, Cullen AP, de Gruijl FR, Longstreth J, Takizawa Y, van der Leun JC. *The human health effects of ozone depletion and interactions with climate change.* Jan 2011. URL:
https://www.ncbi.nlm.nih.gov/pubmed/21253670

Park G, Kim TM, Kim JH. *Antioxidant effects of the sarsaparilla via scavenging of reactive oxygen species and induction of antioxidant enzymes in human dermal fibroblasts.* Jul 2014. URL:
https://www.ncbi.nlm.nih.gov/pubmed/25022355

Sampson S, Gerhardt M, Mandelbaum B. *Platelet rich plasma injection grafts for musculoskeletal injuries: a review.* Dec 2008. URL:
https://www.ncbi.nlm.nih.gov/pubmed/?term=
Mishra+Pavelko+PRP+for+chronic+tendon+2006

Tao S, Justiniano R, Zhang DD, Wondrak GT. *The Nrf2-inducers tanshinone I and dihydrotanshinone protect human skin cells and reconstructed human skin against solar simulated UV.* Oct 2013. URL:
https://www.ncbi.nlm.nih.gov/pubmed/24273736

Wu RT, Cao L, and Mattson E, et.al. *Opposing impacts on healthspan and longevity by limiting dietary selenium in telomere dysfunctional mice.* Feb 2017. URL:

https://www.ncbi.nlm.nih.gov/pubmed/27653523

Yoon HS, Cho HH, Cho S, Lee SR, Shin MH, Chung JH. *Supplementating with dietary astaxanthin combined with collagen hydrolysate improves facial elasticity and decreases matrix metalloproteinase-1 and -12 expression: a comparative study with placebo.* Jul 2014. URL:

https://www.ncbi.nlm.nih.gov/pubmed/24955642

Acknowledgements

We all know the adage "It takes a village to raise a child." What we discovered through creating *Secret To A Younger You* is that it also takes a village to write a book. For us, that village included many of the loved ones and coworkers we see daily, as well as inspiring guides aiding us from a distance.

First and foremost, we must express how grateful we are to our patients. Without their trust and commitment to health, we could not offer the natural cosmetic therapies that led to us writing this book. To "Debbie," we are deeply thankful to her for generously allowing us to tell her story over countless pages. She remains an inspiration to us both and her story reminds us that you, our patients, have the strength to create daily change in your lives.

This book was written under the brilliant guidance of our coach, Angela Lauria. We are deeply thankful to her for the unabashed honesty and imaginative suggestions. She challenged us to develop our own path into authorship and never failed to give beautifully witty, prompt and effective answers to our questions. We give thanks to the insightful author of *Take Back Your Life*, Tami Stackelhouse, who introduced us to Angela.

Every day we are supported by our irreplaceable villagers at Lake Oswego Health Center. The other healthcare providers at the clinic help to make us more knowledgeable physicians by sharing their brilliance with us. Collaborating patient care with these skilled, health-focused individuals leads to better quality care for every individual that passes through the clinic. We are proud and absolutely dependent upon our fantastic office staff and medical assistants who keep us on time, prioritize the concerns and questions of our patients, and make us smile on a daily basis. Our staff keeps our village running smoothly, allowing us to provide safe and reliable care while also focusing on our own professional growth.

To those who inspired us from day one of our careers as prospective physicians and early in our clinical training - our teachers - we are endlessly grateful. This includes our alma maters, Bastyr University and National University of Natural Medicine. We would like to specially thank Dr. Frank Shallenberger who first trained us in medical ozone therapies. His willingness to share his knowledge has helped so many.

To the Morgan James Publishing team: Special thanks to David Hancock, CEO & Founder for believing in our message. To our Author Relations Manager, Megan Malone, thanks for making the process seamless and easy. Many more thanks to everyone else, but especially Jim Howard, Bethany Marshall, and Nickcole Watkins.

A very special thanks and debt of gratitude to both our families. They made it possible for us to expand our already long work days, disappear on countless weekends, and maintain a balance of excitement and calm through the process of writing *Secret To A Younger You.*

ABOUT THE AUTHORS

Dr. Bridghid McMonagle graduated from the University of Washington with a bachelor of science in Environmental Health and a minor in Chemistry. She went on to complete her doctorate from Bastyr University. Dr. McMonagle started to think about a career in healthcare while she was in Thailand during her U.S. Peace Corps service. Living in a small village and 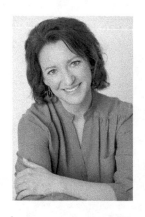 traveling throughout Southeast Asia gave her a new perspective on health. She noticed people had a better sense of community, more time for socializing, and ate simpler foods. After finding her way to naturopathic medicine and completing a residency in Oregon, Dr. McMonagle started her private practice in Lake Oswego. She had no idea how much this would change her life and own health. Thanks to her education, she increased her energy and figured out that her adult acne only happened when she ate gluten-containing foods. Her practice continues to grow and has been very successful. She feels immense joy and gratitude being able to have a job that feels more like a lifestyle. She loves to witness the change in her patients as they evolve into health-minded, inspired, and ultimately healthier people. During free time she loves traveling and exploring other cultures. When at home, you will often find her hiking, running, paddling, or thrashing herself at Crossfit or in a soccer game; they're her versions of meditation!

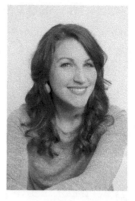

Dr. Kaley Bourgeois is a proud graduate of Portland, Oregon's National University of Natural Medicine (NUNM), the oldest naturopathic program in the United States. She earned her doctorate in under four years as a member of NUNM's first accelerated program after completing a Bachelor's in Exercise Science from Pacific University. Her desire to study and promote natural medicine started in early childhood through the guidance of her mother. Dr. Bourgeois was taught to pursue a healthy lifestyle in order to prevent illness and consider underlying causes before starting a medication. When Dr. Bourgeois later developed an extensive rash with no clear diagnosis and no improvement from prescription medications, she kept faith in what her mother taught. Despite specialists telling her foods were not the cause, she underwent an elimination diet and identified a clear trigger: dairy. Sometimes a simple answer does exist, and when it does not, there is still hope for change. When she isn't seeing patients, Dr. Bourgeois can be found spending time with her husband and daughter, running or baking allergen-free treats that taste deceptively good.

Post-Doctorate Combined Training And Certifications Include:

Bioidentical Hormone Therapy

Fibromyalgia and Chronic Fatigue

Functional Medicine

Intravenous (IV) therapy, including Chelation

LENS Neurofeedback Therapy

Ozone Therapy

Patricia Kane Protocol

Platelet Rich Plasma (PRP) Therapy

Prolozone Injection Therapy

Combined Professional Associations Include:

American Association of Naturopathic Physicians (AANP)

American Association of Ozonotherapy (AAOT)

American College for Advancement in Medicine (ACAM)

The Institute for Functional Medicine (IFM)

Oregon Association of Naturopathic Physicians (OANP)

Physicians Committee for Responsible Medicine (PCRM)

Are you a physician and would like to learn how to incorporate this program into your practice? If so, contact us at (503) 505-9806 for our next professional training.

www.lakeoswegohealth.com

info@lakeoswegohealth.com

Facebook:
https://www.facebook.com/Lake-Oswego-Health-Center-PC-317028868328243/? ref=settings

THANK YOU

Congratulations on finishing this book and taking the time to learn the secret to a YOUNGER AND HEALTHIER YOU! We hope you enjoyed reading this as much as we enjoyed writing it.

As a special thank you to our readers, we are offering 2 free webinars. These are focused on things you can do NOW to make improvements in your skin and overall health.

The first webinar includes keys to improving your nutrition.

1.   Eat Right For Your Skin & Hair

The second webinar will outline how to clean things up and enhance your natural detoxification.

2.   Detox Until You Glow

To access the free webinar, please call our clinic at (503) 505-9806 for directions and password.

For continued up-to-date research articles and health tips, please see our business Facebook page, Lake Oswego Health Center and our website, www.lakeoswegohealth.com.

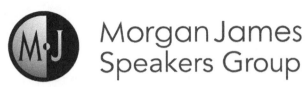

Morgan James
Speakers Group

↗ www.TheMorganJamesSpeakersGroup.com

We connect Morgan James published
authors with live and online events
and audiences who will benefit
from their expertise.

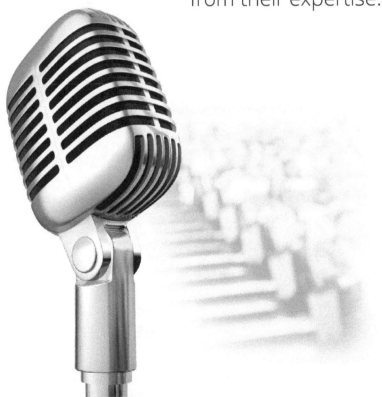